MISCARRIAGE, STILLBIRTH AND NEONATAL DEATH

Guidelines for Professionals

14/1/93.

CONTENTS

It is not easy to give parents whose baby has died the care that they need. It is not easy even for those who are experienced in dealing with bereavement. Yet the quality of care that is given is vitally important. Inappropriate care, or poor management, can be the direct cause of additional trauma for parents. Care that is sensitive and appropriate to parents' needs can help them beyond measure. For although such care cannot diminish their grief, and should not be intended to, it can help them to grieve in the way that they need to, and it can help them, not immediately but later, to accept their baby's death.

These guidelines describe the kind of care which bereaved parents need, and suggest ways in which that quality of care can be achieved.

The guidelines are intended to be used -

- as a source of information and guidance for individual professionals

- as a basis for the formation (or review) of policy for the management of miscarriage, stillbirth and neonatal death and the care given to bereaved parents

- as material for use in training.

It is hoped that the guidelines will be used by all professionals who come into contact with parents who have lost a baby. As well as medical, midwifery and nursing staff both in hospital and in the community, the guidelines should also be of use to other professionals such as social workers, hospital chaplains, bereavement officers, funeral directors, registrars, counsellors, and many others. Each one of these professionals plays an essential individual role in caring for bereaved parents. Their ability to co-ordinate and work together is equally important.

It is emphasised that these guidelines are indeed guidelines and are not intended as a blueprint. Their aim is to promote understanding of a wide range of experiences which, nonetheless, possess important common elements; and to offer a range of strategies for care. Not all strategies will be appropriate in every case and there is a need for sensitivity and judgement in the way the guidelines are applied.

THE ISSUES

It is now time to take stock and listen to the silent grief of mothers who do not dare to rock the boat by a seemingly silly request that society should view her pre-viable fetus as her own special baby.

(The Lancet, editorial, 10 December 1988)

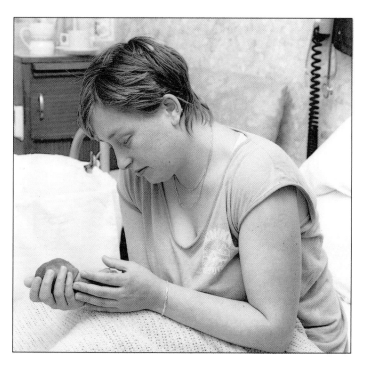

Babies born dead before 28 weeks gestation *

In 1929, when the Infant Life (Preservation) Act set the legal age of viability (in England and Wales) at 28 weeks gestation, very few babies born at earlier gestations survived. Now, over 60 years later, with the same Act still in force, many pre-28 week babies have a reasonable chance of survival.

When these babies do survive, it is of little consequence that they were, in legal terms, non-viable. But when the pre-viable baby is born dead, then problems arise. For while a baby born dead at, say, 25 weeks gestation is, to the parents and to the professionals involved, a baby that could have lived, it remains a non-viable fetus in the eyes of the law and is without legal status.

After a stillbirth, the law requires certain procedures: the stillbirth must be certified and registered; and the baby's body must be buried or cremated. It is also universal practice to obtain parental consent for a post mortem. These requirements, though basic, provide a framework for management. But in the case of the baby born dead before the age of viability, there is no such universally accepted practice. In these circumstances, what procedures are appropriate? How should these deaths be managed?

In recent years, many hospitals have addressed this question and have recognised the need to amend policy and practice to fit the reality of parents' experiences. In consequence, many have now extended and, where necessary, adapted their policies for the management of stillbirth to include

---

* At the time of publication, the age of viability is legally defined as 28 weeks gestation. It is expected that the law will be changed and the age will be lowered in the near future. However, this will not resolve problems to do with the management of loss before the legal age of viability. The issues addressed in this section will remain relevant and the arguments valid.

babies born dead before the legal age of viability. These policies and the experience gained in implementing them have contributed to these guidelines.

Deaths at early gestations

But questions to do with appropriate management do not only apply to those pre-viable babies who might have lived. They apply equally to deaths at earlier gestations, when there can be no realistic expectation of the baby's survival.

Such earlier loss is not necessarily less traumatic. Most women, from the beginning, think of their pregnancy in terms of a baby. If their pregnancy fails, it means, for them, the loss of that baby and of all that that baby meant to them. This is true whether the loss occurs early or late in pregnancy. It is the personal significance of the loss, not the gestational age of the baby, which determines the extent of parents' bereavement and their need to grieve.

It follows from this that the care and support which are offered should be determined not so much by the stage of pregnancy at which the loss occurs as by an understanding of *what the loss means to the parents*. For many parents, an early miscarriage means a great deal, and supportive, sensitive care is badly needed.

This is not to suggest that early miscarriage is the same as later miscarriage or stillbirth, or that it should be handled in the same way. Clearly it is a different physical experience, and its management will differ accordingly. It is also true to say that although early miscarriage can be devastating, it is on the whole less likely to be so than later miscarriage and stillbirth.

But distinctions between one kind of loss and another should be treated with great caution. An early miscarriage may have a meaning which is not immediately apparent. It may, for example, be not the first but the second or third such event for a couple who long for a child. It may cause particular distress because it follows the death of a parent, or because it reopens an older grief or some other unhappiness. Equally, a later miscarriage may be less significant than it appears. A woman who has not invested a great deal in her pregnancy and who has felt from the start that the pregnancy 'wasn't right', may not feel her loss so acutely There may even be an element of relief. There is, in other words, infinite variety of experience and many possible concealed meanings. No easy assumptions can be made about what the loss of a pregnancy means to individual parents.

Comparisons, too, should be avoided. For while professionals are in a position to compare one loss with another and may as a result judge later loss to be greater or 'worse', parents themselves have neither means nor reason to make such comparisons. Each parent experiences, quite simply, the loss of *their* baby. It is not helpful to parents to categorise their experience or grade it in relation to the experience of others.

These guidelines are based on parents' experiences. The experience of early miscarriage is included. For early loss just as for later, the guidelines argue for care which is appropriate to parents' perception of their experience.

The status of babies born dead before the legal age of viability: implications for management

Babies born dead before the legal age of viability have no legal status. Consequently, the law offers no guidance about what may or may not be done with the bodies of such babies. But these babies have a special status in moral terms, having been potential human life. And they have an undeniable status in the minds of their parents. It is therefore essential that appropriate procedures are decided and followed, particularly concerning post mortem examination and disposal.

The experiences of parents make it clear that, as a general principle, the respectful treatment of the baby's body is of the greatest importance, regardless of the baby's gestational age and regardless of the physical reality of the loss (whether baby, fetus or fetal remains). It is clear too that respect is also and equally owed to the parents whose baby it is. These guidelines, therefore, recommend that parental consent should always be sought before any post mortem or other pathological investigation is carried out; and that that consent should be explicit and informed. This recommendation is in line with the 1989 Polkinghorne Report* which states that the mother's consent should always be obtained before an embryo, fetus or fetal material is used for research; that consent should be explicit and positive (as opposed to the absence of objection); and that mothers should be given the information needed to be able to make a proper judgement. (For further discussion, see pages 45-46.)

The guidelines also recommend that, although there are no legal requirements concerning the disposal of the body or remains of a miscarried baby, (that is, no requirement to bury or cremate, as is the case with stillborn and liveborn babies), there should be provision for respectful disposal. What constitutes respectful disposal may vary according to what is lost (especially whether or not there is a body), and more importantly, what is appropriate for and needed by the parents. The parents should be given the opportunity to express their wishes about the disposal of their baby's body, and their wishes should, wherever possible, be respected. This recommendation is also supported by the Polkinghorne Report*. (For further discussion, see pages 67-68.)

* 'Review of the Guidance on the Research Use of Fetuses and Fetal Material' HMSO 1989. The status of this report is made evident in the Department of Health Circular HC(89)23, which requests implementation of the Polkinghorne Code of Practice. In Scotland, see the Scottish Home and Health Department letter to Health Board Managers dated 31 July 1989.

Terminations

It has not been possible in this publication to address the many complicated and special issues which surround the management of termination. It is important to note, however, that the majority of the recommendations made in these guidelines are as relevant for termination as for miscarriage and stillbirth. Special consideration needs to be given to those having terminations for fetal abnormality.

Resources and the implementation of change

Ten years ago, it was felt that parents of a stillborn baby would be best helped if their experience was minimised as much as possible. As a result, many parents did not see or hold their baby, and many were not told what was done with the body. The radical change which has taken place in the management of stillbirth came about because professionals began to acquire a better understanding of what the experience of stillbirth is like and what it means to parents. Equipped with that understanding, they could begin to respond in quite different and supportive ways. Understanding of earlier loss is now also improving. And with it, there is a growing awareness of the common elements which exist in all pregnancy loss. It should therefore now be possible to achieve similar and equally constructive change for the management of miscarriage.

Inevitably, the implementation of change uses resources, and in this case, staff time and training are specially implicated. Yet the improvements brought about in the management of stillbirth and neonatal death have not, on the whole, been costly ones. They are largely the result of changes in policy, and in the style of one-to-one care. The value of such change for parents cannot be over-emphasised.

PRINCIPLES OF

The way miscarriage, stillbirth and neonatal death are managed will vary from one hospital or district to another and from one professional to another. As the many contributions to these guidelines demonstrate, good practice can take many different forms. However, the same *principles* of good practice should apply to any management strategy. Also, though practical care will differ, the same principles should apply regardless of when the loss occurs.

The principles set out below are based on parents' experiences. They describe parents' needs, and suggest ways in which those needs can be met. But good practice is not only a matter of identifying, understanding and meeting patient need. Professionals involved in the management of loss face a task which is extremely demanding - both personally and professionally. So, although parents' needs are of paramount importance, good practice must also take into account what professionals need if they are to be equipped and enabled to care.

Of course, care is provided within a practical framework which, in one way or another, will always impose constraints. Every professional is working within limitations and has to balance what is desirable with what is possible. By describing what is desirable, these principles provide a starting point.

The care given to parents should be responsive to their individual feelings and needs.

All those who are bereaved by the loss of a baby have experiences and feelings in common. But however much is shared, bereavement and grief are also intensely individual. So, while it is helpful if professionals recognise and understand common patterns in parents' experiences, the care and support which they give should be determined by parents' *particular* needs.

It is necessary -

- to avoid assumptions

- to listen and respond to each parent as an individual

- to take account of particular circumstances, particular feelings and beliefs, particular experiences

- to tailor what is said and what is done to the parents/family concerned

- not to be judgemental.

Many parents will be very confused about their feelings and uncertain about what they need. They need an environment where they can discover for themselves what they feel, and where their feelings are accepted. They need to be enabled to work out for themselves what their loss means to them. This process may take a long time and cannot be hurried, so the care parents are given should not

GOOD PRACTICE

pressurise them. Professionals must be prepared to work flexibly, and to the parents' time scale. Professionals must also be prepared to accept that there may be much that parents cannot or do not want to express about the way they feel, and much that an outsider may not be able to understand. This means that it is often necessary to work with uncertainty and to risk making mistakes. What professionals offer will not always be welcomed by or be right for the parents concerned, and although it is difficult, professionals need to be able to tolerate this.

Professionals should be aware that some parents may have special needs. The loss of a baby may, for example, be particularly traumatic for those who have fertility problems, those who have had recurrent losses, those who can have no more children, parents of twins one of whom has died.

Parents need information.

At every stage, parents need and should be given information which is accurate and which is communicated clearly, sensitively and promptly.

In order that they can begin to understand and own their experience, parents need information -

- about what has happened, what is happening or what may happen

- about practical matters, procedures and arrangements

- about the choices which are open to them. They also need clear, factual, unbiased information so that they can make those choices.

It is likely that both parents will need information and it is usually best if it is given to both together.

Information may be supplied in response to questions. No question should be left unanswered. If the answer is difficult for some reason, or even unknown, it is better to admit the difficulty than ignore the question. But parents may also find it hard to put questions into words, or may not know what to ask. So it is helpful to offer information or discussion when the time seems right to do so. Offers should be repeated.

No subject should be avoided. Parents need and appreciate honesty, even if the truth is painful.

It is often hard for parents to take in information the first time it is given and for this or other reasons they may wish to go over it again, and even a number of times. Information should also be available in written form - not as a substitute for discussion but to back it up.

If parents speak little or no English, it is important that they are not denied information for that reason. Interpreters and written information in their own language will be needed.

All professionals in contact with the parents should give consistent information. Parents should not be confused or overwhelmed by being given information by too many different professionals. Co-ordination is important.

Information may also be needed by other family members. But parents' permission should always be asked before talking with others.

Communication with parents should be clear, sensitive and honest.

It is essential that professionals are able to communicate with parents in ways which the parents find acceptable and supportive.

It is helpful if professionals are able -

- to set aside their professional authority when necessary and show a human face

- to talk with parents on equal terms - for example, sitting not standing, and not hiding their own grief about what has happened. Important discussions should not be held while a woman is lying down, unless this really cannot be avoided.

- to use language which is clear, caring and easy to understand. It is important to consider the meaning of words for parents and to avoid unnecessary medical jargon. This means, for example, speaking of a 'miscarriage', never of an 'abortion'; and referring to the baby as a 'baby', not a 'fetus', no matter how small it is. Instead of talking about the 'disposal' of a pre-viable baby, staff might talk about 'what will be done with the baby's body'.

- to be open and honest. Parents would rather know the truth than feel that information is being withheld from them or misrepresented. It is particularly important not to hold discussions in parents' presence which are not shared with them.

- to make time (and show that there is time) for lengthy and unhurried conversations when needed. Even if a conversation has to be postponed, parents will be helped if a firm promise is made to talk later.

- to recognise when a parent does or does not wish to talk.

When the parents do not speak English and the professional concerned is unable to speak fluently in the parents' own language, it is essential that an interpreter is used. (See page 44 for further information.)

Parents should be treated with respect and dignity.

Parents need respect for themselves, for what they have experienced and are experiencing, and for their feelings. The dignity of parents is extremely important at a time when they are vulnerable. This applies equally to both parents: the father as well as the mother.

Demonstrating respect involves -

- recognising the significance of what has happened and therefore not minimising it (for example, not saying "You can always have another baby")

- caring for parents in a way which does not deprive them of dignity. (It is particularly important to recognise that many women find gynaecological procedures both undignified and distressing. Everything possible should be done to minimise this additional distress. For example, women should not be left in the lithotomy position any longer than necessary.)

- treating and speaking about what has been lost, whether a baby, a fetus, fetal remains or products of conception, in a respectful way

- recognising the personal and private nature of grief by caring in a non-intrusive way and giving parents the privacy they need. For many parents, a hospital is an inappropriately impersonal and public place in which to grieve.

enabling parents to participate in the management of their loss. At a time when much is beyond their control, parents need to feel that they have some power over what is happening to them. They should be helped to feel in touch with, and in charge of, their own experience.

Parents' loss should be recognised and acknowledged, their experience and feelings validated.

Parents need others to recognise and acknowledge their loss as part of the difficult process of accepting what has happened. This need, like grief itself, continues over a long period of time.

The expression of sympathy is one important and very simple form of acknowledgement. Neither this nor other ways of acknowledging loss should be omitted because they are painful (although they undoubtedly are). It is more difficult for parents to accept what has happened if people around them appear to deny it.

Parents may also need confirmation of the reality of their experience and reassurance about their responses to it. The loss of a baby at any stage is bewildering and shocking. Parents may struggle to grasp the significance of their experience, to make sense of it in their own terms, and to accept that their feelings are legitimate. Talking about what has happened, going through both the events and the feelings, can be very important. Professionals should make themselves available to help parents do this.

Parents may also need support to do things which will make their experience real to them and create memories for the future.

Parents need to be given time.

The loss of a baby, whether as a miscarriage, stillbirth or neonatal death, often happens with an intensity and speed which make it difficult for the experience to be grasped and understood. In the days, weeks and months afterwards, parents need to overcome shock, understand the experience they have had, and begin to grieve.

Parents need -

- time with each other and/or with their family

- time, if wanted, with their baby

- time to consider and make decisions about practical arrangements

- time in which to re-live, think and talk about what has happened.

Only a very few procedures after a baby's death have to be carried out within a certain time limit (the post mortem examination, for example, and registration - see pages 45 and 50). These should be explained. Parents can then be reassured that there is no other time pressure.

Professionals should try to work to the time scale dictated by parents' feelings and needs. Some parents, for example, who do not wish to see and hold their baby at first, may want to do so later. Some may find that they wish to leave hospital earlier than they had thought, others later.

Sometimes, however, it can be helpful to set time limits for certain decisions. When there is no time limit at all, some decisions (about the baby's burial or cremation, for example) can become much harder to make.

All those involved in the care of bereaved parents should be well informed.

Professionals who are in close contact with bereaved parents and are responsible for their care need to be well informed. They may need to acquire knowledge which is outside their own specific area of expertise.

Professionals need to know -

- their own hospital/community policy regarding the management of miscarriage, stillbirth and neonatal death

- about statutory procedures and practical arrangements

- about what services and support are available to parents locally

- about grief and grieving, particularly in relation to miscarriage, stillbirth and neonatal death.

Professionals need this knowledge in order that they can give accurate and comprehensive information to parents, since only then can parents make informed choices. To be well informed is also important from the professionals' own point of view. Few of those working with bereaved parents have extensive experience of bereavement, and for this and other reasons many do not feel confident. Knowledge can help to give confidence.

   Managers should be aware that a range of other staff will come into contact with parents, such as nursing auxiliaries, ward clerks, domestic staff, porters, receptionists. It is important that they too are informed about policy and good practice.

All those who care for and support bereaved parents should have access to support for themselves.

Professionals whose job it is to care for and support bereaved parents are likely to need support themselves. They too may be very shocked by a baby's death and may need to grieve. They may feel responsible. They may feel unable to cope with either the practical tasks involved or the emotional caring demanded of them. They may find it difficult to manage their personal reactions at the same time as performing a professional role - particularly because the event may bring up emotions to do with their own experiences of loss and bereavement.

The stress involved in the care of bereaved parents is lessened if the professionals concerned -

- receive recognition that their work is demanding and difficult and that they therefore need support, not because of professional inadequacy or personal weakness but as a necessity

- have received appropriate training

- are working within the framework of a clear operational policy

- feel confident that what they are doing or being asked to do is appropriate

- are able to work in co-operation with other professionals

- are given opportunities to explore, understand and express their own feelings - both about bereavement and grief in general and also in relation to specific cases in which they are involved.

Not all professionals will need the same kind or same degree of support. Different options should be available.

PRINCIPLES OF GOOD PRACTICE – SUMMARY

- The care given to parents should be responsive to their individual needs and feelings.

- Parents need information.

- Communication with parents should be clear, sensitive and honest.

- Parents should be treated with respect and dignity.

- Parents' loss should be recognised and acknowledged, their experiences and feelings validated.

- Parents need to be given time.

- All those involved in the care of bereaved parents should be well informed.

- All those who care for and support bereaved parents should have access to support for themselves.

THE GUIDELINES

LOSS OF A BABY AT HOME

It is important to recognise that parents who have lost a pregnancy by natural miscarriage or by a termination of pregnancy may feel as much grief as after a stillbirth or neonatal death, and the period of grief may be prolonged.

(Report of the Royal College of Obstetricians and Gynaecologists Working Party on the Management of Perinatal Deaths, 1985)

This section deals mainly with miscarriage, and particularly the onset of miscarriage which is most likely to occur at home.

Rarely, a baby will be stillborn at home, or die soon after birth following a home delivery. Many of the recommendations made under HOSPITAL CARE: IMMEDIATE AFTERCARE (page 21) and HOSPITAL CARE: POSTNATAL CARE (page 27) are relevant for these deaths.

Some parents choose to bring a dying baby out of hospital so that he or she can die at home. See page 34 for information.

Bleeding in pregnancy / the onset of miscarriage

The first signs of a possible miscarriage can cause women intense and legitimate anxiety. It is important that professionals show that they understand this and treat any sign of an impending miscarriage with proper concern. If a woman contacts her GP, community midwife or health visitor because of bleeding in pregnancy, she should be seen, either at home or at the surgery/health centre, even if she is still in very early pregnancy. Alternatively, a full telephone conversation may be appropriate. She is likely to need -

- preparation for what is happening or may be going to happen

- information about what may be involved (the extent of bleeding, for example, or, for later gestations, labour and delivery) and how to cope

- information about what can or cannot be done to prevent the loss of the baby

- emotional support.

GPs, community midwives and health visitors should be aware that they have a role even when, in medical terms, there may be little they can offer. Miscarriage is unpleasant, undignified and distressing. It is important that women feel supported and cared for.

Miscarriage can involve a lengthy period of time during which parents do not know whether they have lost their baby or not. This uncertainty is hard to bear. So although advice to 'wait and see what happens' is acceptable for a while, the waiting time should be limited by a further appointment or visit, or an appointment for a scan.

Hospital admission for miscarriage

Admission to hospital will be essential for later loss. When notifying the hospital, every effort should be made to secure admission to an appropriate ward rather than the accident and emergency department. See page 19.

For early miscarriage, hospital admission may not be necessary and may be undesirable from the woman's point of view. The hospital environment can change a private and personal crisis into a public and medical event, and for many women this makes the crisis harder to cope with. So the need for hospital admission should be carefully and sensitively assessed. If a woman stays at home, she will need support from her GP and/or midwife.

Feelings after a miscarriage/ the loss of a baby at home

Parents who have lost a baby, at whatever stage in pregnancy or however long after birth, often blame themselves for what has happened. This may be particularly so if the loss has occurred at home. Feelings of responsibility can greatly add to parents' distress. Many will ask themselves, and may also ask the professionals who are caring for them, whether the tragedy could have been avoided if, for example, they had been in hospital or if they had acted differently in some way. Such feelings may be especially acute if the parents chose to have a home birth. It is important to talk about these feelings if parents want and need to, and to answer questions as directly and honestly as possible. Clear information and detailed discussion about reasons for the loss can reduce self-blame and guilt.

I never fail to be overwhelmed by the distress of a miscarriage and it makes me feel very inadequate. I hope that acknowledging this fact is helpful to my patients.

(Dr David Jewell in Tippett S, Jewell D, Masson G, Elphinstone K, *'Bleeding in early pregnancy'*, The Practitioner, 8 November 1989, Vol 233, 1425-30)

HOSPITAL CARE: SCANS

During pregnancy, a woman may be scanned because there have already been indications that something is going wrong. In this situation, she may be prepared for bad news, though she may be hoping for good. Alternatively, a woman may come for a routine scan, assuming that all is well. If she then has to face bad news, she will be unprepared and shocked. In either situation, if the scan is handled well, it can ease the difficult task for a woman of facing up to the loss of her baby.

Recommendations for the management of scans

If a woman is referred for a scan because something appears to be (or to be going) wrong, the scan should be organised promptly (preferably within 24 hours of referral).

A woman should be able to have her partner (or a relative or close friend) with her if she wishes.

The scan should be managed as sympathetically as possible, in a way which will help parents to understand and accept what it shows (even if that is something uncertain). For example -

- the procedure should be explained

- parents should be encouraged to look at the screen and helped to understand what it shows. They may otherwise worry later that a mistake was made, or may simply regret not seeing their baby when they had an opportunity to do so.

- staff should acknowledge that having a scan in order to

Our aim is to establish an approved training syllabus for obstetricians and radiologists, so that in the future every consultant obstetric unit will have at least one expert in obstetric ultrasound to organise, represent and supervise the service, to scan problem cases on a regular basis, to understand the significance of abnormal findings and to recommend appropriate management.

(*Guidelines on training in obstetric ultrasound*, Standing Joint Committee, Royal College of Obstetricians and Gynaecologists and Royal College of Radiologists, February 1990)

confirm an unwanted diagnosis is stressful and upsetting. It can help parents if someone says, for example, 'This must be very hard for you . . .'

Information gained from the scan should be communicated sensitively, clearly and quickly. (See below for further discussion.)

Women may need time to take in and accept the results of the scan and they should be given the time they need. Hospital admission does not normally have to be rushed. Some women, however, having received bad news, find delay difficult and should be admitted as quickly as possible.

The results of scans should be accurately recorded in the medical notes.

Communication of scan information

The most problematic part of the scanning procedure is the communication of the information which is obtained. Parents usually realise when something on a scan is causing concern: their own anxiety (even in a routine scan) means they are particularly sensitive. And since the results of the scan are of such immense importance to parents, they need and deserve to know what has been found as soon as possible. Professionals, on the other hand, knowing parents' anxiety, are themselves extremely anxious not to make a mistake and need time to read the scan and make certain of their diagnosis. They may need time too to find the right words in which to explain what they have seen.

These problems do not, however, justify scanning in silence or unexplained delays in sharing information with parents. It is important that strategies are found to overcome the problems experienced both by professionals and parents.

When a scan is needed because a problem is suspected, it should ideally be managed by a professional specially trained in obstetric ultrasound and able to interpret and impart the scan information. If this is not possible, the scan operator should explain to parents *in advance* that it will not be possible to tell them immediately what the scan shows. He or she should then explain what will happen, who will be involved, and how long it will be before information can be given. Parents are better able to tolerate delay if there is a reasonable explanation for it and if it is time-limited.

If problems are discovered unexpectedly during a routine scan, parents should be told immediately by the scan operator that there is something on the scan which he/she would like to look at more closely or needs a second opinion about. Parents should be asked to wait for the short time needed to interpret the scan and/or find the appropriate professional to speak with them. Again, the length of time should be specified. No woman should be left to wait on her own while another member of staff is fetched. Nor should a woman be sent to another department on her own: a nurse/midwife should go with her.

When giving bad news, it is helpful to bear in mind the significance of the news for the mother / parents. It is vital that what is said is said clearly but gently, that as much detailed information as possible is given, and that questions are answered. The importance of the news should be acknowledged: it is right for staff to express their sympathy and sadness. When a woman's partner is with her, the results of the scan should be discussed with both parents together.

After receiving bad news, women need to be treated with consideration. They may need some time alone, or with a sympathetic professional; they may need to talk over the implications of the scan results. The chance should be offered to make a private phone call to their partner, someone else in the family, or a friend. If a woman is on her own, staff should ask her how she will return home: she may need someone to travel with her.

Always express your sorrow and sympathy and offer what support you can. Parents always remember the way that this sort of news is delivered and the attitude of the people involved.

(Hillingdon Hospital protocol for obstetric scanning)

Amy was told very gently by the scan operator that there was not a heartbeat any more and that he was very sorry. Her husband was with her and they were both shown the screen.

(Extract taken from *Miscarriage* by Christine Moulder, reproduced by kind permission of Pandora Press.
© 1990 Christine Moulder. All rights reserved)

Scanning after miscarriage

If a woman is referred for a scan after a miscarriage, when she knows that she has lost her baby, the recommendations above are still relevant. In addition, the scan operator should be aware that it may be a particularly unhappy experience to attend for a scan along with women who are still pregnant; and that, although parents may know that their pregnancy has ended, the results of the scan should be handled no less sensitively.

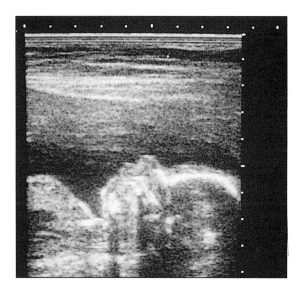

HOSPITAL CARE: MISCARRIAGE / LABOUR AND DELIVERY AFTER A DEATH IN UTERO

A stillbirth can never be a joyful event, but sensitive, confident midwives can make labour and delivery a positive and successful experience for parents, and for themselves.

(Mallinson G, *When a baby dies* Nursing Times, 1 March 1989, Vol 85, No 9, 31-4)

This section makes recommendations for the hospital management of miscarriage, and of labour and delivery after a baby has died in utero. The way staff implement these recommendations will vary slightly according to their assessment of what is appropriate in each case, and according to the timing of the loss.

It is crucial that miscarriage (at any stage of pregnancy), and labour and delivery after a death in utero, are managed well. Poor hospital care can greatly exacerbate parents' distress, both short and long term. Parents do not forget the events surrounding the loss of their baby and need to be able to remember an experience which, however distressful, was handled with care and sensitivity.

Preparation for labour

In some circumstances, it is possible to discuss the process of miscarriage or labour and delivery in advance. The woman may want her partner to be involved in this discussion and this can be important for him. By talking beforehand, parents can feel prepared for and better able to face what is going to happen.

Honesty and clarity are important: women need to know what to expect. Many are surprised and shocked to find that even a relatively early miscarriage is akin to labour. A woman late in pregnancy whose baby has died in utero may not anticipate a 'normal' labour and delivery. Those in their first pregnancy may not know what a 'normal' labour and delivery is and may need a lot of information to prepare themselves.

Women may have particular fears about what they will deliver. Preparation for this is needed too. If there may be abnormality or maceration, or if it is unlikely that there will be a fetus, this should be gently explained.

Choice

Women should be given as much choice as possible about, for example, pain relief, position, holding the baby straight after delivery or later, or in the case of earlier miscarriage, seeing what they have lost (see 'When there is no body', page 24). Information is needed to make these choices.

Information and explanation

Throughout, women need to be given clear information about what is happening, and what is likely to happen, in language which they can understand. Events, decisions, procedures should all be explained, and where there are uncertainties, these should be admitted. If a woman is aware of what is happening and can understand it, she will be better able to keep pace with the experience and will feel more in control.

Questions should be welcomed and encouraged. There may also be questions parents need to ask but find difficult to express.

It is important that fathers are fully and clearly informed. They are likely to feel worried and fearful for their partner, seeing her distressed and probably in pain. They may also feel very helpless. Information, reassurance and involvement are all helpful.

Unacceptable and unnecessary medical terminology should be avoided. See page 10 for more information about communication.

Support

If a woman wishes, she should be able to have her partner (or a close relative or friend) with her throughout. This should apply at no matter what stage the pregnancy is ending.

Whether or not she will have her partner with her, she needs to be reassured that staff will also give her support.

Most mothers did not blame their doctors for their baby's death, nor did they expect their doctors to say something to make them feel better. They wanted them to explain in simple language what had gone wrong, and then to listen and accept their distress.

(Forrest GC, Standish E, Baum JD, *'Support after perinatal death: a study of support and counselling after perinatal bereavement'*, British Medical Journal, 20 November 1982, Vol 285, 1475-9)

Although some women, in certain circumstances, may actually prefer to be alone (though knowing that they can get help when needed), others do not wish to be alone at any time - and should not be so.

Where a woman should be cared for

The place in which a woman is cared for during a miscarriage or stillbirth affects how she manages her loss, and how she feels about it both at the time and afterwards. In an inappropriate place, women can feel that they are abnormal and unimportant, that their experience is denied, that staff do not understand the personal significance of the event. Ideally, women should be admitted to a ward -

- where they are expected

- where the care of women either miscarrying or delivering a stillborn baby is part of the planned work of that ward

- where staff understand the significance of what is happening, and have the training / experience to provide appropriate practical and emotional care.

It is likely that different hospitals will meet these criteria in different locations. In each hospital there should be agreed guidelines to determine when care should be on the gynaecological ward, when on the labour ward.

If the labour ward is used and it is certain that the baby will be born dead or cannot survive, unnecessary technological equipment, such as monitoring and resuscitation equipment, should be taken away.

It is not appropriate for a woman to miscarry in the accident and emergency department. If a woman has been referred to hospital by her GP, the GP can notify the hospital and in most cases it should then be possible for the woman to bypass the accident and emergency department and be

When talking to parents they invariably mentioned the distress they felt when hearing the crying of babies delivered in other labour rooms. This led us to devise a policy to deliver mothers with known fetal death in utero on Delivery Suite 2, ... Relatives are invited to use the sitting room next to the delivery room. This eliminates the stressful situation of having to share the waiting area with parents who are expecting a happy event.

(Bhattacharjee C, *Improving the care of bereaved parents'*, Nursing Standard, 21 February 1990, Vol 4, No 22, 18-20)

admitted to an appropriate ward. Women who are admitted through accident and emergency should be transferred to a ward as quickly as possible. At no time should a woman who is miscarrying be left on a trolley in a public place.

Induction

Some parents benefit from a delay between receiving confirmation that their baby has died and induction. Where there is no risk in delay, 24 or 48 hours' space can give parents time to accept the diagnosis and collect their thoughts about the delivery (and loss) to come. Some may prefer to wait longer and see whether labour begins naturally. Other parents feel that to carry a dead baby or continue with a non-viable pregnancy for any time at all is intolerable and will need to be admitted as quickly as possible. It is important to discuss options and give parents the information they need to make the decision that is right for them.

Induction should be explained in advance. Women need to know what will happen, and what the experience may be like.

Pain relief

Pain relief options should be talked over very carefully both before and during miscarriage/labour, with pros and cons explained.

Used well, (that is, in a way that suits the feelings and needs of the individual), pain relief can help women to feel more in control of what is happening. There is a risk, however, that pain relief may diminish a woman's sense of participation in her experience. She may also feel, later on, confused about events which she needs to understand. So it is important to find the appropriate level of pain relief for each woman.

When assessing what pain relief will be helpful, it should

be remembered that shock and misery may mean that pain is felt more acutely; and that pain relief may be needed even for early miscarriage.

ERPC (Evacuation of retained products of conception)

Once a miscarriage has been confirmed, some women will want an ERPC as soon as possible; others will need time to take in the news. If possible, women's sense of timing should be respected.

Explanation and preparation are important before an ERPC. The woman should know what will happen, what will be done, and why it is necessary. She should be prepared for some bleeding afterwards, and possibly cramps - for which pain relief should be offered.

Although in medical terms an ERPC is minor and routine, it is a significant and often worrying event for the woman, and probably for her partner too. It marks the end of pregnancy in a very definite and final way and afterwards there can be intense feelings of sadness and emptiness, even if there is also relief that the miscarriage itself is over. So it is important that professionals recognise and acknowledge the significance of what is happening.

It is essential that what is removed at an ERPC is explained to the woman both before and after the operation. Otherwise she may fantasise about what has been removed. It may help some women to see what has been removed and this option might be offered.

HOSPITAL CARE: IMMEDIATE AFTERCARE

This section deals with the care needed by parents immediately after a miscarriage or stillbirth, or after a very early neonatal death.

The care that is given will be very different when there is no body. But professionals should be aware that in these circumstances loss may still be acutely felt and appropriate care is needed.

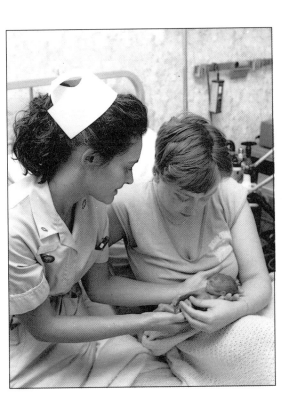

Telling the parents and other staff about the death

When a baby dies during labour / delivery or immediately afterwards, parents should be told at once.

All staff who are involved and all who might be involved must be promptly informed about the death. Besides medical, midwifery and nursing staff, this includes the hospital social worker, hospital chaplain, physiotherapist, administrative staff, nursing auxiliaries, domestic staff and others who may come into contact with the parents.

For communication between hospital and community, see page 26.

Medical certification

A baby should be certified as having been born alive if there are any signs of life at all, even near the limits of viability. The parents will then have a proper birth certificate and death certificate for their baby. For further information about certification, see page 48.

Seeing and holding the baby

Parents should be encouraged to see and hold their baby. If they do not want to do this immediately, the offer should be kept open for them and repeated. They should not be pressed to do what they feel unable to do but must know that they are free to change their minds and can ask for their baby to be brought to them whenever they feel ready.

Some parents want to see and hold their baby but need help to do so. It may be helpful -

- to wash the baby and carefully wrap him or her

- to lay the baby in a cot beside the parents so that they can

Careful management helps to preserve the dignity and poignancy of the experience and to initiate the difficult process of mourning.

(Bourne S, Lewis E, *'Pregnancy after stillbirth and neonatal death'*, The Lancet, 7 July 1984, 31-33)

As you died a couple of days before you were born, the doctors considered you to be just under 28 weeks. This meant no birth or death certificate - as if you didn't exist. That still hurts.

(A parent - SANDS Newsletter, Autumn 1986)

be with their baby but can take time before they hold him or her

- if a member of staff holds the baby first and stays with the parents for a while

- to show the parents a photo of their baby first, and perhaps talk about it

- to keep the baby in a nearby room for a while. It can be easier for parents to ask for their baby to be brought to them if they know he or she is not far away.

When there are twins or more babies, it is important that parents can see and maybe hold both or all their babies together. Otherwise it is difficult for parents to grasp the reality of what has happened. Later, the memory of being with both or all their babies together can be valuable.

When abnormality is visible or there is maceration, parents should be gently warned of this. Maceration should be explained. It can help if the baby is wrapped in a blanket and parents look first at the baby's normal, perfect features. Parents who are anxious about looking at their baby will need help and support (see suggestions above).

Seeing and holding their baby is important for parents no matter how small their baby is. It may sometimes be hard for staff to treat a tiny baby of, say, 12 to 15 weeks gestation in the same way that they would a larger, more developed baby. But parents do not compare their baby with others. It is important that all babies are handled respectfully and lovingly. For very tiny babies, washing and wrapping may not be appropriate. It is most natural to hold these babies in the palm of the hand.

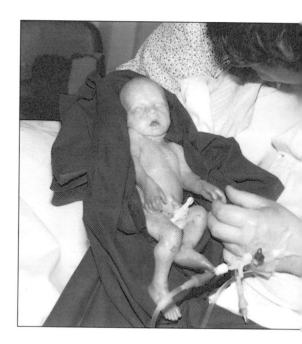

I would have liked to have held my daughter. I don't think anyone would have objected, but then again nobody offered her to me.

(Helen whose baby was stillborn)

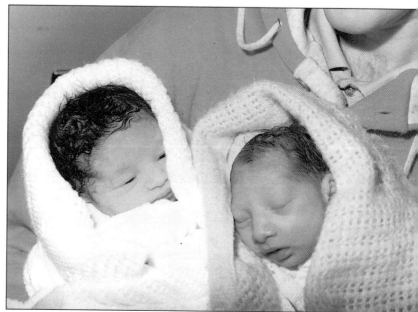

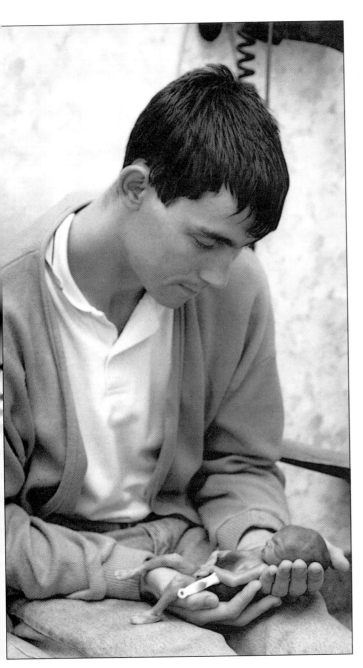

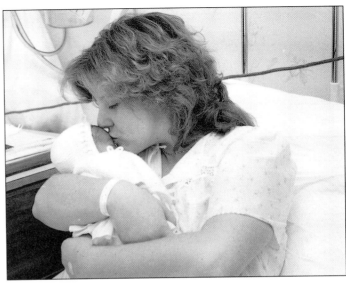

The young doctor asked if we would like to see Philip but we declined the offer - a decision I will regret to my dying day. If only someone could have talked to me, could have explained how important it was to say goodbye to our baby, could have told me how it would help with the grieving process, could have just gently taken me by the hand and supported me.

(Anne, whose baby lived for one week)

When there is no body

When there is no body, women may still want and need to see what they have lost. If they do not see it, they may later become anxious and upset, and may imagine something far worse than reality. So the option of looking at the products of conception / fetal remains should be offered, and the offer repeated if necessary. Staff should be prepared to explain what the products/remains are, and to answer questions.

It may be particularly important to explain why there is no recognisable baby. Most women think of their pregnancy, from the beginning, in terms of a baby and it can be hard to reconcile what was, for them, an emotional reality with the physical reality of the loss.

Parents should be told what will happen to the products / remains (see page 68 for information about disposal).

Time alone, and time with the baby

Parents should, when they are ready and if they wish, be left alone and in privacy, although they should know that staff are available if needed. Parents should be able to keep their baby with them if they wish. A cot should be available for the baby.

Parents may want to dress their baby in clothes they have brought. They may need help to do this or may want to ask someone to do it for them. Some hospitals provide clothes, including very tiny ones, in case parents have none. Or the baby might be wrapped in a shawl.

Some parents may want prayers to be said, or their baby to be blessed, perhaps by the hospital chaplain or by their own minister. Staff should offer to contact whoever is needed. Sometimes parents want the staff who have been involved in their baby's delivery to be involved in a religious ceremony. (See also RELIGIOUS BELIEFS AND PRACTICES, page 41.)

Parents may need to spend a long time with their baby and they should not be hurried. They should not be asked to part from their baby before they feel ready to do so. They should then be reassured that their baby will be safely kept for them for a stated period of time, that the body will not deteriorate, and that they can ask to see their baby again if they wish.

Parents may still want private time with their baby even if the baby is very tiny. No matter how small, the baby should not be taken away from the parents without their knowledge.

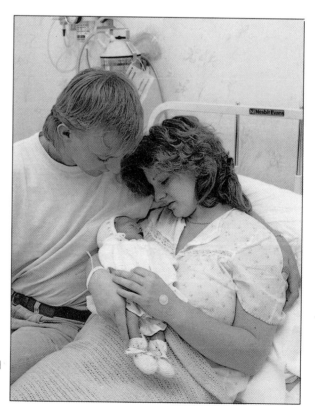

We were allowed to stay in the delivery room for as long as we wanted, and it was up to us when we wanted to say 'goodbye' to Naomi and hand her over to the staff. Peter, Naomi and I were left on our own and the staff just popped their heads round the door occasionally to see if we needed anything. They really got the balance between helpfulness and privacy exactly right.

(Sue, whose baby lived for 20 minutes)

Storage of babies' bodies

Before the baby is taken to the mortuary, the body should be labelled with the mother's name and hospital number, date and time of birth and death, the baby's sex and other details, including the baby's name if there is one.

Babies' bodies must be properly stored so that if parents wish to see their baby again, they can do so without distress. Each hospital should have a policy which states how, and for how long, babies' bodies should be kept, and this policy should be known to medical, nursing and mortuary staff.

All babies' bodies should be kept, regardless of gestational age. Although it is the practice of some hospitals to store small bodies in formalin, refrigeration is preferable so that parents can see their baby again if they wish.

For information about funerals/disposal for babies born dead before the legal age of viability, see pages 67-68.

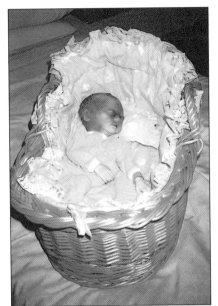
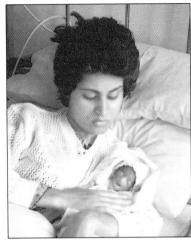

Photography

Soon after delivery, a number of photographs should be taken especially for the parents.

Polaroid photographs provide parents with something immediately but fade over time. Copies of polaroid photographs can be made by most film processors and these will not fade, but the quality is poor. Good quality photographs on 35 mm film should also be taken.

Parents may want to choose how the photographs are taken and may want several different pictures. Their baby might, for example, be photographed in their arms, in a moses basket and/or on a blanket. They may want photographs of their baby dressed, or naked, or both. They may prefer black and white photographs to colour. The photographs will be of immense importance to parents over the years and it is extremely important to try to meet their requests and take high quality pictures. There may also be cultural or religious factors which dictate how parents will want the photographs to be taken.

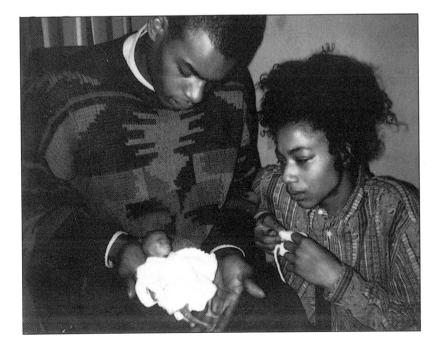

When there is a multiple birth, even when one baby has survived and one has died, parents may want to have a photo of their babies together. They will not otherwise have any record of the complete reality of their experience. This can be important, so if parents do not think of it themselves, it might be suggested to them.

Parents may also want to take photographs themselves and this too might be suggested. Their own photographs should be in addition to those taken by the hospital. Some hospitals provide cameras in case parents do not have their own.

If parents do not want the photographs, they should be filed with the medical notes. The parents may ask for them weeks, months or even years later. Parents should be told that the photographs will be kept and that they can ask for them at any time.

Photographs should be taken of every baby, no matter how small or how early the gestation. When there is abnormality, or the baby is macerated or damaged in some way, it is possible that parents will not want to keep (or even see) the photographs, however carefully and sensitively they are taken. But it is important not to make assumptions about parents' wishes.

If an outside film processor is used, it is important to check that they understand the value and nature of the photographs they are developing.

The medical record

A complete and accurate record should be made in the medical notes and the front of the notes should be clearly marked in some way to show that the baby has died.

The information that is recorded should be passed to community staff (see opposite) and should be available at the follow-up appointment (see page 37). At that appointment, or later, parents may want to ask questions or may express worries which only factual information can answer.

Communication with community staff

It is essential that community professionals are promptly informed of any miscarriage, stillbirth or neonatal death. It should be the allotted task of one member of the hospital staff to pass on this information. Parents themselves should never have to break the news or be visited by a professional who does not know what has happened. The GP and others must be equipped with information which will enable them to answer questions and give the kind of physical and emotional care that is needed.

The community professionals whom it is appropriate to contact will vary. The woman's GP should always be informed, and possibly her community midwife and health visitor. They should be informed -

- by telephone, within 24 hours, with a confirmatory letter to follow

- and subsequently by letter, giving a full history. This detailed information should be sent as soon as possible. Post mortem / investigation results (if applicable) should be sent later.

Community staff should know whom they can contact at the hospital in order to obtain information.

If the family doctor is to give good and sensitive care to the family, he needs to be aware of the event. We inform him by phone initially and follow this up with a brief letter. A full summary then follows in due course. We do the same with the health visitor - a phone message, then a brief form, and a later summary.

(Neonatal Unit, University College Hospital, London)

HOSPITAL CARE: POSTNATAL CARE

The recommendations given here are for postnatal care following miscarriage, stillbirth and neonatal death. What is appropriate will vary according to individual need and circumstances.

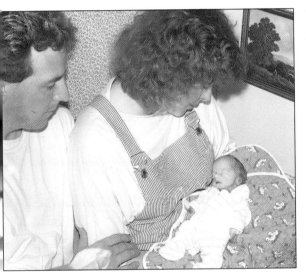

Choice of ward or room

If possible, women should be offered a choice between a single room or a ward. Privacy is essential for many, but some women prefer to be with others. For example, some women who have miscarried relatively early in pregnancy find that it helps them to be with others who have had similar experiences.

In some hospitals, a special parents' room is available for those whose baby has died or is very ill.

A bed should be provided so that a woman's partner, or a relative or close friend, can stay with her through the night. It is important that partners are made to feel welcome.

Medication

Although analgesia may be very helpful, most women are not helped by taking sleeping tablets. If a woman asks for sleeping tablets, or if it is thought they may be of help, her needs should be carefully assessed. It may be helpful to talk with her and gently explain that no medication can take away her grief, and that sometimes medication can get in the way of feelings which are important and necessary.

Lactation

Lactation is one of the most distressing physical symptoms that a woman can experience after losing a baby. Her breasts may be swollen and throbbing, and may also leak milk. It can be a constant, painful reminder of her baby's death, and unfortunately emotional distress may increase the flow of milk. Sympathetic support is essential as well as practical help to suppress the milk and to feel as comfortable as possible.

The management of lactation varies. In some hospitals, drugs are routinely prescribed; elsewhere they

The family room is in fact a suite comprising a double bedroom, a private bath / shower room and a completely furnished lounge. It has been tastefully decorated throughout, taking away much of the hospital atmosphere . . . The basic idea is to give bereaved parents an element of privacy and the ability to be together at a time when couples need each other. It also gives the facility for close family and friends to be able to visit.

(Solihull Maternity Hospital)

are avoided. Milk may be gently expressed to ease discomfort, but care should be taken not to over-express as this will stimulate and increase the milk supply. A good supporting bra can help, and cold compresses to reduce swelling and pain. Women may also need pain relief.

It may be some time before lactation stops altogether. Individuals vary, and the stage of pregnancy or age of the baby is obviously a factor, but women may continue to produce milk for several days, and it may be between 2 and 4 weeks before discomfort ends. It is best if women are prepared for this.

A woman may lactate or leak small amounts of milk even after an early miscarriage at, say, 3 months of pregnancy. This is more likely if a woman has breast fed before.

Parents' access to their baby

Parents should have access to their baby. They need to know whom they should speak to if they want to see their baby.

Parents who did not hold their baby after delivery may want to do so later and should be given encouragement and help if needed (see page 21).

Parents should never have to go to the mortuary: their baby should be brought to them, somewhere where they can be private and comfortable. This might be a room on the ward, quiet room, or mortuary chapel. The baby should be dressed, and carried in, for example, a moses basket. Staff may need to explain to parents beforehand that their baby will feel cold and rigid, but can be touched and held. If the baby is wrapped in a shawl, holding will feel more natural.

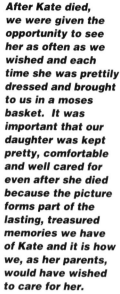

After Kate died, we were given the opportunity to see her as often as we wished and each time she was prettily dressed and brought to us in a moses basket. It was important that our daughter was kept pretty, comfortable and well cared for even after she died because the picture forms part of the lasting, treasured memories we have of Kate and it is how we, as her parents, would have wished to care for her.

(Lynn, whose baby lived for 10 hours 35 minutes)

If parents want to see their baby after he or she has been taken to the mortuary, the midwife will collect the baby in the moses basket and take the baby to the sitting room where parents and relatives can have as much time with their baby as they would like. The midwife will then take the baby back to the mortuary.

(*Stillbirth - Caring for bereaved parents*, Christa Bhattacharjee, 1989)

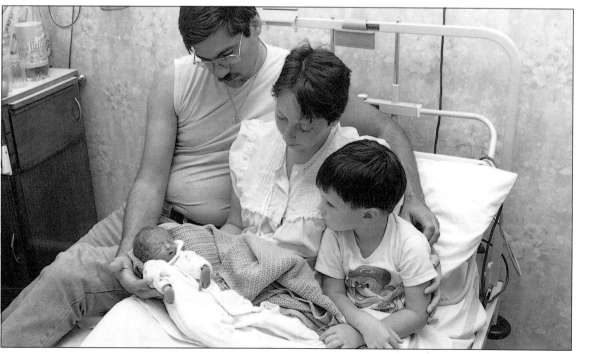

Naming the baby

Parents may want to name their baby (if they have not already done so). Once they have decided on a name, some may want the hospital chaplain, or another religious adviser, to give a blessing or say prayers for their baby by name.

Staff should ask parents whether they may use the baby's name. If there is no name, then it is important to speak of *your* baby, (or 'little one' or any other affectionate term). 'The' baby is very impersonal.

Naming can be important, even for parents who have had an early miscarriage. It helps to give a focus to ideas about the baby. It is easier to choose a name if the baby's sex is known and this should always be recorded if it is possible to tell. But parents may still want to give their baby a name even if it is impossible to know the baby's sex.

Creating memories

Parents may want to gather mementoes such as their baby's cot card, name band, locks of hair, foot or hand prints, stills from scans, a fetal monitor tracing, their baptism card, and so on. They will value anything which will help them to remember their baby.

Parents should be asked before a lock of hair is cut or a foot or handprint taken.

The pictures of our baby form the mainstay of our memories. Along with the cards and letters, the wristband, the footprints the midwife made us, the post mortem report, even the receipt for the funeral . . . These, more than the ashes from the cremation, are the remains of our baby.

(Naomi, whose baby was stillborn)

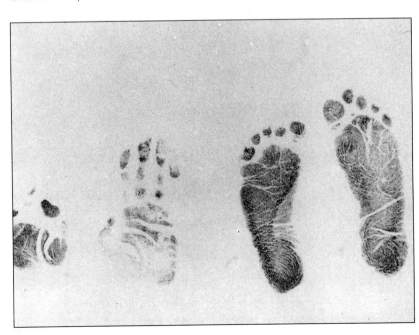

Deciding about a funeral or ceremony

Many parents will want to make arrangements for a funeral or some other kind of ceremony for their baby. Others will be pleased if this possibility is suggested to them. They will need information to help them plan what is right for them. See FUNERALS, BURIAL, CREMATION, page 61.

Staff should be aware that parents who have lost babies at very early gestations can be helped by holding a funeral, or by a service or ceremony (see pages 67-68 for information).

Involvement of other members of the family

Parents may want other members of the family, including other children, to see the baby. It is almost always helpful for siblings to see their dead brother or sister. What is imagined is often frightening: the reality can be reassuring. It can also help later if the family has shared memories to talk about.

Visiting hours, if normally restricted, should be extended so that the family can be together. If the parents are not in a separate room, they will need somewhere private and quiet where they can be with their family. Some hospitals have a bereavement room, or quiet room.

Parents may wish to take photographs of their baby with others in their family. Photographs taken of siblings with their dead brother or sister can be helpful later, especially if they are very young at the time the baby dies. The hospital might offer to take these photographs.

Talking, listening, counselling

Parents may need to talk at length and in detail about the pregnancy, the miscarriage/labour and delivery and all the circumstances surrounding their baby's death. They may

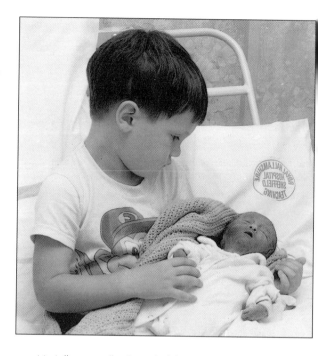

want to talk generally about their hopes and expectations for the child and the dreams they had for him or her.

Visitors, if wanted, can be helpful as listeners and staff too should try to give time for listening. It can be especially helpful if staff who were involved in the miscarriage/delivery are available because they can confirm what happened as well as answer important questions.

The hospital social worker and/or other professionals trained in counselling should also be available.

The hospital chaplain should be notified if parents wish. Staff should offer to contact anyone else whom parents may want to see.

In some hospitals, after a baby's death, one member of staff takes on the main care of the parents. This means that parents have someone to whom they can relate, and someone to whom they can address their questions and requests. They do not have to repeat conversations with a number of different professionals, and can feel more secure.

However, this does place a heavy responsibility on the member of staff concerned who needs to have some support. See SUPPORT FOR PROFESSIONALS page 74.

Repeated offers/suggestions

Although parents should never feel pressured, it may be appropriate if certain offers and suggestions are gently repeated. For example, if they have not already done so, parents might be encouraged to see and/or hold their baby, to give a name, to take photos or gather other mementoes (see pages 21,25 and 29). If they have at first rejected the idea of a funeral or other ceremony, they may want help to reconsider this and be sure of their decision.

Information and discussion

Parents will need information about -

- the post mortem or other laboratory investigations (see page 45)

- certification and registration procedures (see page 48)

- funerals, burial, cremation, or disposal (see page 61)

Written information should also be given (see 'Written information', page 32).

Parents may also need to talk and ask questions about -

- physical symptoms, such as bleeding, lactation/painful breasts, painful stitches

- their chances of having a live, healthy baby in the future. Discussion about a possible future pregnancy will probably be most appropriate when the results of a post mortem or

other tests are available, but staff should not postpone discussion completely. It is important to respond to what is likely to be a major anxiety. Staff should honestly explain that what can be said, for the time being, is limited, and should be careful not to speculate or present possibilities to parents as though they are facts.

- the timing of a future pregnancy. Parents need to be aware that, before conceiving again, they will first need to grieve for the baby who has died. They also need to know that the anniversary of their baby's death is likely to be a difficult time. If their next baby is born at about that time, they may find the pregnancy and the birth itself very distressing. For most parents, it is helpful if the timing of their next pregnancy is totally different to the one which has just ended unhappily. All parents need to be able to make their own informed decision.
  If appropriate, parents should be given information about how they can obtain genetic counselling and/or advice on preconception care.

- when they should (or have to) go back to work. It is not necessarily best for a woman to go back to work as soon as possible. Many need more time to recover than they (or others) anticipate. Some (perhaps especially women who have had miscarriages) may need to understand that time may be needed for emotional as much as physical recovery.

- anxieties to do with going home. All parents need to know about the services and support available once they are at home (see 'Leaving hospital', page 32, and CARE AND SUPPORT AT HOME, page 55).

- contraception. Many parents will not want to think about sex at this time, others may want and need to make love for the comfort it can bring. It is important that advice about contraception is offered tactfully. Discussion about preventing pregnancy can seem insensitive when parents are mourning the loss of their baby.

Length of hospital stay

If there are no overriding medical reasons, the woman herself should decide the length of her hospital stay. Some women benefit from a longer hospital stay because it gives them time and rest which they would not have at home. It is important that women do not leave hospital before they feel ready to do so.

Some women find the prospect of leaving hospital difficult. Arrangements for support from community professionals can help. See 'Leaving hospital', below, and CARE AND SUPPORT AT HOME, page 55.

Leaving hospital

Before a woman leaves hospital -

- she should be given a follow-up appointment for 4 to 6 weeks time (see page 37).

- she should be given information about the services and support, both professional and voluntary, which will be available to her once she is at home (see 'Written information', opposite). Contact should be made with the appropriate community professionals (see 'Communication with community staff', page 26). A visit from the community midwife, if appropriate, before a woman leaves hospital can help to bridge the gap between hospital and home care. Some hospitals are able to arrange for home visits from a member of the hospital staff, such as a social worker.

- she should be given a phone number so that she can contact the staff who have cared for her after leaving hospital

- any outstanding antenatal / scan appointments must be cancelled. This is often forgotten and causes parents unnecessary distress. It should be the designated task of one member of staff.

Written information

Although verbal explanations and opportunities to talk are important, parents also need written information.

Hospitals should provide parents with written information about -

- procedures and practical arrangements (certification and registration, funeral arrangements etc), with the names, addresses and telephone numbers of relevant professionals.

- services and support (professional and voluntary) available to them on leaving hospital. Information should include, if possible, the roles, names and telephone numbers of community professionals; the names and addresses of national and local support groups/organisations (see page 78), and local contacts.

Specific local information is particularly helpful. The task of registration, for example, can be made a great deal easier if parents are given information not only about what to do but also the register office address, the registrar's name, and office opening hours.

Women who have miscarried should be given written information about the causes of miscarriage in general, the physical and emotional aftermath, going back to work, and trying again. This information is particularly important after miscarriage because the hospital stay is likely to be short.

Many hospitals now produce their own leaflets giving both general information and also specific information about local arrangements and services.

Parents may also appreciate suggestions about books they might find helpful to read. See SOURCES AND FURTHER READING, page 77.

In areas where there are ethnic minority populations, written information should be prepared in appropriate languages. This material should be developed with members of the relevant community: simple translation from an English version is unlikely to be successful. Additional information may be necessary, or changes may be needed to accommodate cultural differences.

HOSPITAL CARE: NEONATAL UNITS

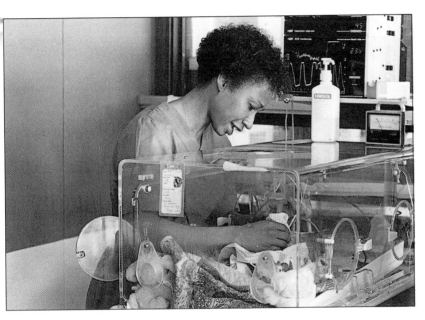

When the decision was taken to stop treatment we were given a pleasant, quiet room in which to hold and be alone with Kate. Our families were allowed to come and go as they pleased and our minister was able to come and baptise our daughter.

(Lynn, whose baby lived for 10 hours 35 minutes)

When a baby is known to be dying

When a baby is known to be dying, the parents should be told immediately. They then need to be involved as much as possible in the care of their baby and should be able to stay overnight in the hospital if they would like to do so.

If possible, parents should be able to move, with their baby, into a separate, private room. They may wish to dress their baby in his or her own clothes. The neonatal unit should have clothes available in case they are needed. They may wish to take photos (see Photographs, page 35). They should be encouraged to ask for help with anything they find difficult to do.

It is important that the father is as much involved as the mother. The parents may also want others in the family, such as other children and grandparents, to see and be with the baby.

Parents need privacy during this time but they should not feel isolated. If their baby continues to live for some hours, there may be questions they need to ask, and they may need support and reassurance. They need easy access to one or two professionals who can provide continuity of care.

It is unlikely that parents will have seen anyone die before and they may feel frightened. They may need to know what it may be like for their baby, though some will find it difficult to ask. They may also need reassurance that their baby can be made comfortable.

When a decision has to be made to withdraw life support, parents should be involved in this decision and may need to talk about it. Some parents will want to continue life support - and their decision should be respected.

Parents may wish to hold a religious ceremony - Christian parents, for example, may want to have their baby baptised. Parents should be asked what they would like, and staff should offer to contact whoever is needed and to help with arrangements. It is important that parents are given privacy to hold whatever ceremony they choose. Some may wish staff to take part.

Taking a dying baby home

During Mark's terminal illness . . . I think we are more grateful than anything that we could keep Mark at home. Because Mark came home, all his possessions and clothes were his.

(Amanda, whose baby lived for 2 weeks)

It may be possible for parents to take their baby home. No matter how caring the staff, hospitals remain impersonal and public places, and it can be very important and helpful for parents to be with their baby in a private and familiar place, even if only for a short time. It can also be helpful for others in the family, especially older brothers or sisters.

Some parents will be clear that they want to take their baby home and will feel confident about doing so. Others may need encouragement and reassurance. For some parents, it will not be an appropriate thing to do.

Parents are likely to need emotional and practical support from both hospital and community staff. Hospital professionals should liaise with community staff before the parents leave hospital to ensure that appropriate support is available.

Some parents will be helped by taking their baby out of the neonatal unit, at least for a short time. For example, they may want to take their baby into the hospital grounds for a short time. They can then feel that their baby has experienced more than just the hospital environment and has been a part of their world.

When a baby dies

Before death if possible, or immediately afterwards, all apparatus should be removed so that parents can hold their baby.

Parents who are alone with their baby when he or she dies are likely to need confirmation of the death. They should be able to contact a member of staff when they need to do so.

If parents are not present when their baby dies, they must be told of the death in person and as soon as possible. There is no hurry to certify the time of death and in some cases it may be possible, in the parents' interests, to delay certification until after they have had some time with their baby.

Afterwards

After their baby's death, parents should be able to be alone with their baby in quiet and privacy for as long as they wish. There should be a room available where they can be comfortable and undisturbed, and where there is a baby nest/moses basket available so that they can put down their baby if they want to. Parents may also want to be with their other children or relatives.

Parents may want to be visited by members of staff who have cared for their baby. It can help to mourn with those who have been most involved in their baby's life. This can also be helpful for staff.

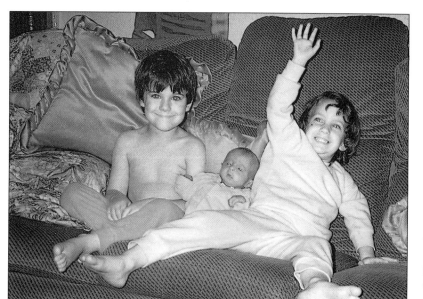

It is important that parents are helped to do all that they want to do for their baby. Staff can make suggestions, and should offer to do for parents (or with them) what they would like to do but cannot manage for themselves. For example, parents may want to -

- wash their baby (or help, or watch this being done)

- dress their baby in special clothes

- collect mementoes of their baby, such as a lock of hair, foot and hand prints, the cot card, weight and measurements, and so on

- take photos (see opposite)

- put a small toy or something else that is personally significant into the moses basket with their baby

- ask the hospital chaplain or their own minister to give a blessing or say prayers for their baby

- take their baby home for a while, or keep the baby at home and make their own funeral arrangements (see page 63).

A baby should only be taken to the mortuary when the parents are ready. They should be reassured that their baby will be safely kept for a stated period of time, that the body will not deteriorate, and that they can ask to see their baby again if they wish. For information about the storage of babies' bodies, see page 25.

When a baby dies at a hospital distant from the parents' home, the hospital should arrange for the baby's body to be transported back to the parents' home area.

Photographs

Photographs of the baby should be taken before death, if possible, and also after death and given to the parents. Parents may also want to take their own photographs and this might be suggested to them if they have not thought of it. Some hospitals provide cameras for parents to use if they have not got their own. See page 25 for further information about photography.

Staff on the neonatal unit who have got to know the baby and parents well may also want to keep a photograph of the baby.

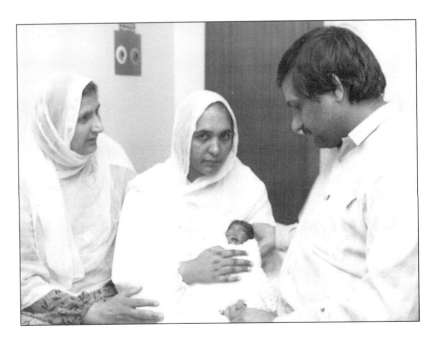

Information for parents

Parents will need information about -

- the post mortem (see page 45)

- certification and registration (see page 48)

- funerals (see page 61)

- services and support available both in the hospital and outside, professional and voluntary (see page 55)

Parents should also be given written information to take home (see page 32).

Parents should be given copies of any forms which they sign. They will value any memento of their baby's life, no matter how official. They may also need to reassure themselves about what they signed: sometimes it is hard to recall what is done at a time of stress and this can cause unnecessary worry afterwards.

Leaving hospital

Before leaving hospital, parents should be given opportunities to ask questions and talk at length with appropriate staff about anything that concerns or worries them (see page 31).

A follow-up appointment should be arranged (see opposite).

Maintaining contact with parents

It can be important for parents to remain in touch with the unit where their baby died. When they leave, they should be assured that they can contact or return to the hospital during the coming weeks and months. A named contact within the unit might be offered to parents - perhaps a nurse, social worker, hospital chaplain, or doctor who has been involved with the parents during their baby's time in hospital.

It can be helpful if hospital staff have some continued contact with parents after they have left the hospital. At least one follow-up appointment is essential (see opposite), but in addition, a phone call or home visit, if the parents agree, from a member of the hospital staff can help parents to feel that their baby is still thought about and that their grief is recognised.

Many neonatal units now have a book of remembrance in which parents can make an entry if they wish (see page 73). They may not be ready to do this until some weeks after their baby's death.

Many units send letters or cards to parents on, for example, the anniversary of their baby's death.

An annual remembrance service for all babies who have died on the unit can give parents the chance to meet with others who have had similar experiences and can give staff the opportunity to share in parents' grief. It can also be a time to re-establish friendships which were cut off by the baby's death.

Our important connection with the SCBU did not end after Jason died, the support continued and we were especially touched when so many nurses came to Jason's funeral. We have since been back to visit Jason's 'home' many times.

(Joanne, whose baby lived for 11 days)

HOSPITAL CARE: FOLLOW UP

(See also CARE AND SUPPORT AT HOME, page 55.)

Arrangements for follow up

Before a woman leaves hospital, a follow-up appointment should be arranged for 4 to 6 weeks time. It should be explained what the appointment is for and what will happen. Parents should also know that they can get in touch with the hospital before this appointment if they need to do so. They should be given a number and the name of a person to contact.

Parents should be encouraged to come together to their follow-up appointment: it can be just as important for the father as for the mother. Some women may want to bring a close relative or friend.

Parents should be encouraged to write down questions and worries in advance and bring their list with them.

It can be very distressing for parents who have lost their baby to attend postnatally along with other mothers and babies, or to attend an appointment held in the antenatal clinic or neonatal unit. If possible, a separate time and place should be found.

When a member of staff has been closely involved in a woman's care (her midwife, for example) or perhaps in the care of her baby (on the neonatal unit), it can be helpful if he or she can also come to the follow-up appointment. Not only the parents but also the professionals may welcome this renewed contact.

Women who have lost a baby, at whatever stage or for whatever reason are never seen back in antenatal clinic - they either go to a gynae clinic or to see the consultant in his/her office for post-delivery follow up.

(Southmead Hospital, Bristol)

The need for follow up after miscarriage

It is essential that a follow-up appointment of some kind is offered to all women who have lost a baby, however early in pregnancy.

Women who miscarry early can have a great need for information and discussion about why the miscarriage occurred and whether it will happen again. These needs cannot always be met by an appointment with the GP or by the kind of hospital follow up usually offered after early miscarriage. Some hospitals are experimenting with alternative arrangements, such as a miscarriage clinic run by a senior nurse/counsellor, a follow-up group run by a nurse, or follow up by a community midwife. However, there will always be some women (and not only those who miscarry repeatedly or late in pregnancy) who will need a follow-up appointment with a sympathetic doctor and the means should be found to provide this. Hospital and community should have a co-ordinated approach to the care and follow up of women who miscarry at early gestations. This should ensure that everyone is offered follow up that meets their needs. (See also CARE AND SUPPORT AT HOME, page 55.)

At the follow-up appointment

At the appointment -

- the woman's medical notes must be available. They should be clearly marked in some way so that all staff are aware of the reason for the visit.

- if there has been pathological investigation, the results should be available (see page 48)

The professional(s) involved should be prepared and able

to provide detailed information and answer a wide range of questions as honestly as possible. Adequate time should be allowed as there is likely to be a great deal to discuss and much will be difficult and emotional.

Discussion should cover -

- how the woman is now feeling physically, and how both parents are feeling emotionally

- what happened and why (even if no reason is known). See THE POST MORTEM / LABORATORY INVESTIGATIONS, page 45.

- possible future pregnancies. Referral for investigations/medical help may be needed, particularly for women who have suffered recurrent miscarriages. Genetic counselling may be appropriate and this should be explained and an appointment offered. If parents do not want genetic counselling immediately, they will need to know how they can contact the service if and when they want to.

- information about sources of professional and voluntary help and support (see CARE AND SUPPORT AT HOME, page 55). Parents should be clear about how to obtain what they want or need, either now or in the future.

At the end of the appointment, parents should be told whom they can contact if they have further questions, problems or worries. Some hospitals offer a further optional appointment after about 3 months.

Professionals should be aware that parents often have very high expectations of the follow-up appointment. They may come to it hoping for clear answers and reassurance, and often neither can be provided. The way the appointment is conducted is therefore very important. It is helpful if the professional(s) involved can speak clearly, honestly and sympathetically. They should acknowledge parents' loss and grief. (See page 10 for information about communication.)

Checklist for hospital staff (to be used after miscarriage, stillbirth or neonatal death)

This is an example of the kind of checklist which can be used in hospitals to ensure that important procedures are not overlooked. Individual hospitals may need to add to or adapt the list to suit their own practice.

Mother's name

Address

Home phone number

Father's name

Other children

name	age

Baby's name

LOSS NOW

	weeks gestation
miscarriage	
stillbirth	
neonatal death	

PREVIOUS LOSS

	Date
miscarriage	
stillbirth	
neonatal death	

	TICK	SIGN	DATE
Mother informed of death by			
Father informed of death by			
Baby seen by mother			
Baby seen by father			
Baby held by mother			
Baby held by father			
Baby seen/held by other relatives			
Photos taken of baby			
Photos offered to parents			
Photos put on file			
Mementoes offered to parents -			
stills from scan			
cot card			
name band			
lock of hair			
foot/hand print			
other			
Chaplain or parents' own religious adviser notified (if desired by parents)			
Baptism or other religious ceremony offered			

		TICK	SIGN	DATE
Consultant obstetrician informed				
Consultant paediatrician informed				
Appropriate worker informed -				
social worker				
maternity liaison sister				
bereavement counsellor				
Parents given opportunity to discuss their baby's death with -				
senior doctor				
midwife				
nursing sister				
GP informed	by phone			
	by letter			
Health visitor informed	by phone			
	by letter			
Community midwife informed				
	by phone			
	by letter			
Consent for post mortem requested				
Consent given / refused				
If refused, other investigations requested				
Consent given / refused				
Post mortem form completed and signed by both parents				
Preliminary post mortem results explained to mother and father				

	TICK	SIGN	DATE
Death or stillbirth certificate completed, explained and given to parents			
Certificate for baby born dead before the legal age of viability offered to parents			
Certificate accepted/put on file			
Information given on when and where to register stillbirth, birth and death.			
Information on funeral arrangements given and discussed			
Parents' decision -			
Hospital: burial / cremation			
Private: burial / cremation			
Chapel service explained requested/not requested			
Parents told about book of remembrance			
Parents given -			
hospital/unit parents' booklet			
SANDS parents' booklet			
Mother given information about suppressing lactation			
Parents seen by consultant or senior staff prior to discharge			

	TICK	SIGN	DATE
Local support groups telephone number given -			
SANDS			
MISCARRIAGE ASSOCIATION			
TAMBA			
SATFA			
Other			

Would parents like a group member to contact them?   YES / NO

Hospital contact:

Name

Telephone number

Post natal follow-up appointment date

clinic sister notified

Genetic counselling appointment (if appropriate)

COPIES OF THE CHECKLIST CAN
BE OBTAINED FROM SANDS

RELIGIOUS BELIEFS AND PRACTICES

When a baby dies or a pregnancy fails, religious beliefs and practices may be, or may become, particularly important for some parents. Religious faith may offer some degree of comfort, hope and explanation for the loss. The religious practices and ceremonies surrounding death may also give parents and families a formal and traditional way of expressing their shared grief and of honouring the life that has been lost. It is clearly very important that professionals who are caring for grieving parents show respect for the parents' religious beliefs and practices.

Each religion offers different insights into the meaning of life and death. Each religion ascribes different significance to life in the womb and so to stillbirth, miscarriage and neonatal death, and may attach different ceremonies to them.

However, sets of 'facts' about different religions and the provision that should be made when a family of a particular religious group is bereaved, are often unhelpful to professionals, even if it is possible to compile them. In attempting to set down theological and practical 'rules' for different faiths, it is easy to oversimplify and distort beliefs and practices that are complex, subtle and individual.

In addition, many religions make little or no formal provision around miscarriage, stillbirth and neonatal death, and there may be no clear authoritative rulings on what should be done. Many faiths do not have a hierarchical authority structure whose role it is to give such rulings. For many families private, informal, individual religious observances are most important.

Despite all this, it is clearly right that staff should be equipped with some basic understanding of what is and is not likely to be acceptable to bereaved parents of different faiths and of how to find out what each individual would like. They are more likely to feel able to ask sensitive questions about what parents would like if they know the basic framework within which they are working and what kinds of questions might be insensitive. Wherever possible they should be equipped with a general understanding of the religious faith of the parents they are caring for and should know at least if there is anything that is likely to give offence.

To achieve this, each hospital needs to develop and maintain contacts with members of local religious communities and to discuss with them the possible preferences and practical needs of parents of that community whose babies die or are miscarried. Where possible a network of personal contacts should be developed to whom professionals can turn for sensitive help and advice as needed. The hospital chaplain and the local Community Health Council and Community Relations Council may be able to help with the initial contacts.

Hospital chaplains

Hospital chaplains can be a source of comfort and counselling for bereaved parents of all religious beliefs and of none. Many hospital chaplains will hold simple services in the hospital chapel for parents of any religious beliefs, and also for parents who have no clear religious faith but who want a formal funeral service for their baby.

Hospital chaplains can also help provide information and advice for staff, both about Christian denominations other than their own, and about non-Christian groups. As mentioned above, they may also be able to provide local contacts with different religious groups.

The needs of bereaved parents

Whatever religious affiliation - or none - is entered on a mother's notes, it is wisest not to make assumptions as to what observances parents may wish to make when their baby dies. They should therefore always be asked tactfully and sensitively what their wishes are and every effort should be made to put them into effect.

This may mean -

- listening to parents if they wish to discuss religious issues

- asking sensitively whether they would like some kind of religious observance or ceremony at the birth or death of their baby and helping, where necessary, with any arrangements and with contacting appropriate people.

For members of some religious groups it is likely to be important to organise the funeral within 24 hours of the baby's death. Parents may need help with getting the medical certificate and other certificates signed as soon as possible (see page 50 for more information). These parents often miss out on the contact and continuing support normally offered by hospital and community staff in the time between the death of a baby and the funeral, and to miss out on the opportunity to say goodbye to staff, for example in a neonatal unit. Staff may need to make a particular effort to contact these parents at home in the first few weeks so that they do not feel cut off.

- ensuring that the shrouds, chapel fittings, remembrance and sympathy cards and anything else that the hospital uses do not offend or exclude non-Christian parents.

- checking whether other assumptions of British hospital practice, based largely on Christian beliefs and practices, may be inappropriate. For example, ministers of religion do not have a pastoral role in all religions. They may not visit the sick and the dying and it may be inappropriate to call on them to do so. There may be other people in the community whom the parents would like to give them support. Parents' religious views may influence who should wash and handle their baby. Taking a photograph of a baby with flowers may sometimes give offence.

CARING FOR FAMILIES OF DIFFERENT COMMUNITIES

Everybody has a culture. That culture influences what they regard as normal, reasonable, acceptable. It influences, for example, their reactions to birth, death and bereavement, and affects how they begin to understand and cope with them.

People who share a culture are more likely to see things in the same way. So professionals who share their clients' culture may feel more confident about offering comfort and support, even in very difficult situations such as the death of a baby.

Caring for people whose culture is to some degree different can be much harder. It is not possible to rely on shared meanings and reactions, and it is less certain what people need or will find helpful. Cultural factors on both sides become a barrier to mutual understanding. Professionals can often feel de-skilled, inadequate and frustrated.

In these circumstances, it is tempting to turn to 'experts' or books for help and information. But generalised information about groups or communities can be inaccurate and misleading and should be handled with care. In addition, all cultures are constantly going through a process of change. And most individuals within minority groups in Britain will also be influenced to some degree by both their own culture and that of the majority community. Some things will be important to each person and others will mean little. It is impossible to tell what matters to any bereaved parent except by asking.

The following principles may be helpful for professionals working with bereaved families whose cultures they do not share:

● Even more than usual, it is important to find out from the parents themselves what they want and what they would find helpful. People do not usually mind being asked personal questions provided they are asked in a respectful and sensitive way.

● Professionals' own cultural assumptions may be inappropriate when working with families of other communities. For example, in many cultures, pregnancy and childbirth and everything associated with them are traditionally women's responsibilities. Some people may prefer or expect husbands to be excluded. On the other hand, formal and public religious events, such as funerals, may involve mainly men. Although circumstances and personal preferences may mean that this pattern no longer holds for many couples in Britain, it will be true for some. Female relatives may sometimes be more important than the husband in supporting a bereaved mother. Their role should be acknowledged and supported.

● Some standard NHS routines and practices to do with, for example, washing and laying out a dead baby may be offensive to members of minority cultures. It is important to be sensitive to this and to try and be flexible about procedures whenever possible.

● Reactions to death and bereavement have strong cultural influences. For example, the way that people express grief, their physical reactions and behaviour at times of great sorrow, whether they feel that it is acceptable to cry loudly in public, how people less closely involved with the death should show their sympathy, and so on, may differ a good deal. Free expression of grief can cause problems in the confined spaces of a hospital. If grieving family members are genuinely distressing other families, it may be advisable to try to find them a side room or an office.

● Doing things in the correct or familiar way can become particularly important when somebody dies. Staff need to find out if there are any important religious or other rites that the parents want to observe and help them arrange these if necessary.

● Any information gathered about, for example, the likely needs and attitudes of a particular community, should always be checked out with a reliable person from the community concerned. Class, age, gender and other differences should be borne in mind as with the white British community.

● Professionals should not believe, still less base their practice on, negative generalisations about minority communities. British attitudes of racial and cultural superiority make these particularly common. Every culture is equally valuable and makes sense in its own terms. If some feature of a culture seems senseless or extraordinary, it has been misunderstood. It is important to find out more.

● Members of minority communities are less likely to be familiar with the procedures that surround a death in Britain and may need particular explanation and help in dealing with practical matters such as registration, organising a funeral etc.

● As always, the most important thing is to try to give support and care that is appropriate to each individual.

INTERPRETERS

A professional interpreter

Good communication is, if possible, even more important when caring for bereaved families whose culture is unfamiliar. When there is also a language barrier, professionals are likely to find it impossible to give good care. It is essential that they have access to good interpreting support, preferably a professional interpreter who -

- is trained and experienced

- is fluent both in English and in the parents' mother tongue

- understands the medical terminology involved

- understands grief and grieving and the principles of good care and support

- can help the professional understand how he or she can be most effective in caring for this family, and can help sort out possible areas of misunderstanding and confusion in both directions

- will help ensure that the parents get the information and support they want

- is acceptable to the family and will maintain confidentiality.

Using children to interpret

After a baby's death or the loss of a pregnancy it is never acceptable to use a child of any age to interpret.

Using adult family members and friends

Using an adult family member can also be problematic. Family members are often called upon to interpret because their English is better than anyone else's, but it may still not be good enough for the sensitive and difficult communication required with bereaved parents. In addition, family members may be too distressed to interpret everything that is said, or may want to protect the parents from its full impact. Relationships within families are often complicated, and the parents may not be happy to discuss their personal worries and grief or intimate medical details through another family member. In some cases they may not be sure that what is said will be kept confidential. All the above applies also to adult friends.

Hospital lists

Many hospitals have a list of bilingual staff members who may be called upon to interpret. Such lists can be useful but only if very carefully used. The members of staff on the list must be truly bilingual and must all be professionals. It is not acceptable to use non-professional staff to interpret in this highly charged and difficult area. Parents must be able to trust the confidentiality of what is discussed and revealed, and the interpreter must be able to deal with the subject professionally and accurately, without embarrassment or distress, while supporting and listening to the parents. Parents who speak little or no English are likely to need more, rather than less, professional help and support. It is also not acceptable from the point of view of the non-professional staff, to ask them to take on the burden of interpreting in this or any other difficult or distressing situation.

Other arrangements

Those hospitals that do not have their own full or part-time professional interpreters should contact their local councils or local adult education department for interpreters. Sessional interpreters will need briefing well and a good deal of support over the days and weeks in which they are involved with the family.   All staff should have easy access to information on how to contact interpreters for the main local languages.

THE POST MORTEM / LABORATORY INVESTIGATIONS

Reasons for pathological investigation

Parents themselves may request a post mortem / investigation and if they do, it should certainly be carried out. This applies regardless of the baby's gestational age.

Alternatively, doctors may wish to suggest a post mortem / investigation to parents in order that they have as much information as possible about the cause of their baby's death. Even if no definite cause can be found, parents may benefit from knowing that the death has been thoroughly investigated.

Pathological investigation may also be desirable for scientific reasons and some parents are helped by the knowledge that a post mortem examination of their baby will be of benefit to others as well as themselves.

Parental consent

Parental consent is required for a post mortem on any baby stillborn after the legal age of viability* or any liveborn baby who subsequently dies.

In the past, consent has not generally been obtained for post mortems / investigations on babies born dead before 28 weeks gestation. However, the status of these babies in moral terms and also in the eyes of their parents is no different, and much distress can be caused to parents who

* At the time of publishing these Guidelines, the age of viability is legally defined as 28 weeks gestation. It is expected that this will be lowered.

discover belatedly that a pathological examination has been carried out without their knowledge. So parental consent should always be obtained, regardless of the gestational age of the baby. This recommendation is in line with the recommendations of the 1989 Polkinghorne Report (see page 7).

If, after discussion, parents do not want a post mortem / investigation to be carried out, their wishes should be respected.

When asking parents for their consent, professionals should be prepared to talk with them at some length, explaining the reasons for it and what is involved, and responding to parents' worries about the procedure. Discussion should be unhurried, honest and intended to help parents reach the decision which is right for them. The person who talks with the parents should be senior, and well informed. He or she needs to be able to understand parents' possible misgivings.

Parents from some religious groups may be reluctant, or find it impossible, to agree to a post mortem / investigation. Some may be able to give their consent if they can be reassured that the procedure will not delay an early funeral, and that it will be carried out with due care and reverence.

Whenever possible parents should be asked for their consent together, and both should sign the consent form if they wish to do so. A duplicate copy of the consent form should be offered to the parents.

Deaths reported to the coroner / procurator fiscal

If there are any suspicious circumstances or uncertainties surrounding the cause of death, the doctor must report the death to a coroner (or in Scotland, a procurator fiscal).

The coroner may decide to order a post mortem to try to establish the cause of death. This does not normally delay the funeral and it should be possible to repair the body well enough for the parents to see their baby again afterwards (see 'Repair of the body', opposite). If the parents wish to object to the post mortem for any reason, they should telephone the coroner's office immediately since coroner's post mortems are usually done as soon as possible. The coroner or one of his officers can be contacted 24 hours a day. If the coroner decides to go ahead with the post mortem despite the parents' objections, he has the legal right to do so. However, the parents can, if they wish, apply to the High Court to try to stop the post mortem.

The coroner does not normally give parents a copy of the post mortem report but will usually send one to the hospital consultant concerned. The hospital should offer the parents the chance to discuss the post mortem findings.

(See pages 53 for registration procedures following a coroner's post mortem.)

In Scotland there are no coroners but the equivalent duties are carried out by a procurator fiscal.

Parental consent: information for parents

Many parents wish to discover a reason for their baby's death but feel anxious about giving their consent for a post mortem / investigation because it is such an invasive procedure. It will help them to make their decision if they are given clear information about -

- why it is thought that investigation is necessary and would be valuable (and so why consent is being sought)

- the possible outcome of the examination. Parents need to know that although it *may* provide a definite cause of death, an indecisive result is also possible. They also need to know that even if the post mortem / investigation does not identify a clear cause of death, it can still provide valuable information. It may, for example, rule out causes which have been suspected and maybe feared. Or it may provide information relevant for a future pregnancy.

- where, when and by whom the examination will be performed. For many parents, particularly those who have lost a recognisable baby and so have a body to treasure, consenting to a post mortem involves 'handing over' what feels to them to be, and indeed is, a part of themselves. They need to know where their baby will be, for how long, and when they can have access to the body again.

If the post mortem is to be carried out at another hospital, the body should not be transferred to that hospital until the day of the post mortem and should be returned as quickly as possible after the examination. This applies as much to babies born at early gestations as to those born later.

- when, to whom, and how the results of the post mortem/investigation will be made available. See 'Results' page 48.

- what will happen to their baby's body / remains after the post mortem, (see 'Repair of the body' and 'Disposal' below). If parents wish to know exactly what will be done to their baby's body, they should be told.

Parents who do not consent

Some parents will refuse to consent to a post mortem and it is important that this is accepted and their wishes are respected.

No pressure should be put on parents, under any circumstances, to consent to a post mortem which they do not want. However, for some parents it may be appropriate to explore possible alternatives to a full post mortem. For example, parents may agree to a post mortem provided that the baby's head is not touched. They may be able to accept investigation which is limited to a particular system, such as the heart or kidneys. Or they may agree to needle biopsy of the organs.

Repair of the body

Perhaps the strongest and most difficult feeling which parents have about a post mortem is fear of the damage which will be done to their baby. This feeling cannot be ignored and professionals must be prepared to discuss it with parents in whatever ways seem most helpful.

With good practice, it is possible for the baby to be restored and carefully dressed so as to be acceptable to the parents to see again after the post mortem. The restoration of babies of early gestations is more difficult and can be time-consuming but it is not impossible and is certainly desirable.

It is important to explain to parents, as gently as possible, what will and will not be possible after the examination. For example, if a hospital's practice in restoring bodies means that it is not possible for parents to hold their baby once a post mortem has been carried out, then parents must be warned of this before they give their consent. Parents who wish to see their baby again after the post mortem should be told about the incisions which are made: they must not discover the stitching by accident.

It can be suggested to parents that they might provide clothes, including a bonnet and shawl, for their baby to be dressed in after the post mortem. Hospitals should, however, have clothes available (including very small ones) in case parents do not wish to do this. Alternatively, if there is to be a privately arranged funeral, parents can ask their funeral director to prepare their baby for them.

Disposal

When parents have decided not to have a funeral and have asked the hospital to dispose of their baby's body/remains after the post mortem, it is important that this is done in a respectful way. When discussing the post mortem beforehand, parents should be given the opportunity to express their wishes about the disposal of their baby's body and their wishes should, wherever possible, be respected. See FUNERALS,BURIALS,CREMATION, page 61 for more information.

[Repair of the baby] is done by the post mortem technician. In my hospital it has the highest priority and a baby may be viewed or even picked up after post mortem and repair.

(Dr Gillian Gau, Queen Charlotte's and Chelsea Hospital, London.)

The request form for laboratory investigation on the baby / fetus should be clearly marked with the parents' wishes for disposal.

Maternity Unit (South Cleveland Hospital)

Results of the post mortem / investigation

Parents will be anxious to receive the post mortem / investigation results as soon as possible. There should be the minimum of delay in providing parents not only with the results but also with the opportunity to discuss them fully.

An appointment should be made for the parents to come, together if possible, to discuss the results with the obstetrician and/or paediatrician who have been responsible for their care. When both an obstetrician and paediatrician have been involved, they should liaise and agree whether one or both should see the parents. In some cases, it can be helpful for the parents to speak to the pathologist.

The professional who is talking with the parents should be prepared for a wide discussion. For parents, the pathology results may raise many issues which it is important for them to discuss. One issue, in particular, may be the possibility of another pregnancy.

If the baby's death is found to be the result of a genetic disorder, parents should be offered the opportunity to see a genetic counsellor. They may want to take up this offer at a later date when they feel ready for it, so they should know whom to contact and how.

If there are indications that further investigations or treatment would be necessary in a future pregnancy, parents must be told how this can be organised.

In some hospitals, parents are given, or at least offered, a copy of the full pathologist's report. Elsewhere they are given a summary. The full report should be sent to the parents' GP. Parents should be told whom they can contact if they have any further questions.

CERTIFICATION AND REGISTRATION

Medical certification

Babies born dead before the legal age of viability*

When a baby is born dead before the legal age of viability, the law does not require the birth to be certified or registered.

However, parents who decide to hold a funeral for their baby will need a certificate or letter from the doctor or registered midwife who attended the delivery, stating that their baby was born before the legal age of viability and showed no signs of life. (For an example of such a certificate see opposite.) Funeral directors will not accept a body of any gestation for cremation or burial without documentation. The person who issues the letter or certificate should explain the contents to the parents.

Apart from their practical function these letters or certificates are valued by many parents as a formal recognition of their baby's existence. All parents should also be offered a copy to keep, whether or not they plan to hold a funeral.

Note: In Scotland a baby born dead after 20 weeks may be registered as stillborn if the parents wish, provided the doctor who attended the delivery issues a medical certificate as outlined opposite (see also page 51). The doctor is under no legal obligation to issue such a certificate.

* At the time of publication the age of viability is legally defined as 28 weeks gestation. It is expected that this will be lowered.

Certificate for a baby born dead before the legal age of viability

This is to certify that

_____

was born to _____ (mother)

and _____ (father)

on _____

after _____ weeks gestation

and showed no signs of life.

Signed _____

Name _____

Registered qualifications_____

Date _____

Stillbirths

When a baby is stillborn, the doctor or registered midwife who attended the delivery, or who examined the baby's body after delivery, gives the parents a Medical Certificate of Stillbirth (in **Northern Ireland** a Certificate of Stillbirth). This must be taken to the registrar of births and deaths for the stillbirth to be registered (see page 51). The doctor should explain what is written on the certificate to the parents. Many parents also appreciate being offered a copy to keep.

If the baby is to be cremated, the doctor who verified the stillbirth fills in a cremation form. Only one medical signature is needed and no fee should be charged for it. (In **Northern Ireland** a second medical signature is required.) See page 53 for coroner's / procurator fiscal's cases.

Neonatal deaths

When a baby dies within 28 days of birth, having been born alive at whatever gestation, the doctor who attended the baby must give the parents a medical certificate. In **England and Wales** this is a Special Medical Cause of Death Certificate (full legal name, Medical Certificate of Cause of Death of Live-Born Children Dying within 28 Days of Life). In **Scotland** and **Northern Ireland** an ordinary Medical Cause of Death Certificate is used.

This certificate must be taken to the registrar of births and deaths for the baby's death to be registered (see page 52). The doctor should explain what is written on the certificate to the parents. Many parents also appreciate being offered a copy to keep.

Although both the baby's birth and death must be registered, parents do not need a document from the hospital to register the birth. The health authority will already have informed the local registrar.

If the baby is to be cremated, the doctor who verified the death and signed the certificate signs the cremation form. A second medical signature is also needed. The doctors may waive the fees for this. See page 53 for coroner's / procurator fiscal's cases.

Registration

All live births, all deaths, and all stillbirths must be registered in person, ie, not by letter or telephone. The person or people registering the death must take the certificate issued by the doctor (described above) to the register office.

Registration must normally take place before the baby can be buried or cremated (but see also 'Urgent burials' below).

Urgent burials

If the death or stillbirth occurs on or just before a weekend or public holiday, and it is necessary for religious reasons that the baby is buried as soon as possible, the local registrar will normally issue a Certificate of Burial to allow the funeral to go ahead. (This is not possible for a cremation or if the death needs to be reported to the coroner.) Formal registration can take place later, up to 14 days after a neonatal death and up to six weeks after a stillbirth. (In Scotland, registration can take place up to eight days after a neonatal death and 21 days after a stillbirth.)

Seeing the registrar

The legal procedures and forms involved in registering a stillbirth or a neonatal death are not, in general, the way that parents would like them to be. Registrars are bound by many inflexible and outdated laws and regulations. Even so, the certificates issued to the parents give formal recognition to their baby's existence and are important documents.

Parents find it helpful when registrars recognise both how difficult and how significant it is for them to register their baby's death. Some parents may appear calm because they are still in a state of shock and disbelief. Some may find the process of registration an intrusion into their private grief. All parents can be greatly helped if they are treated with kindness and respect, and if their loss is sympathetically acknowledged. They may also need advice from the registrar on how to get the best they can out of the registration system.

It is helpful for registrars if hospitals write 'death of a young child' in the corner of the envelope containing the medical certificate. The registrar can give the parents special consideration as appropriate, for example, seeing them first, or keeping them apart from parents registering new births.

Hospital responsibilities

The bereavement officer or another member of the hospital staff should make sure, before the parents go to the register office, that they have a general understanding of what will happen there, that they have the medical certificate and the other information the registrar will need, and that they know what they can ask for at the register office to ensure that the certificates issued are, as far as possible, as they wish. The parents may like someone from the hospital to go with them to the register office.

If there are likely to be any problems, for example, delay due to the mother's illness, or complications with entering the father's name in the register because the parents are not married, one of the parents or, if they prefer, a member of the hospital staff, should telephone the registrar for advice.

Where to register

In England and Wales all deaths and stillbirths must be registered in the registration district in which they occurred. (This may not be the registration district in which the parents live.)

In Scotland and Northern Ireland, deaths and stillbirths can be registered either in the registration district in which they occurred, or in the registration district in which the person registering the death usually lives (providing he or she lives in Scotland or Northern Ireland respectively).

The bereavement officer or another member of the hospital staff should give the parents the address of the register office with details of how to get there and, if necessary, a map.

Babies born dead before the legal age of viability*

In **England**, **Wales** and **Northern Ireland**, babies born dead before the legal age of viability cannot be registered.

In **Scotland** a baby born dead after 20 weeks gestation may be registered if the parents wish, provided the doctor who attended the delivery or examined the baby's body after delivery issues a medical certificate (see above). The doctor is under no legal obligation to issue such a certificate. The registration procedure is as described below.

* At the time of publication the age of viability is legally defined as 28 weeks gestation. It is expected that this will be lowered.

Registering a stillbirth

A stillbirth should be registered within six weeks (21 days in **Scotland**) and cannot be registered after three months.

See page 53 for coroner's / procurator fiscal's cases.

People who can register a stillbirth

The registrar will normally expect the baby's mother, or, if the parents are married, either parent, to register the stillbirth. If the parents are not married but the father wishes to register the stillbirth by himself, or to have his name entered in the stillbirth register, he should contact the registrar for advice on the necessary procedures.

If neither the mother nor the father can register the stillbirth, contact the registrar for advice.

Information the registrar will need

The date and place of the delivery (and the time in **Scotland**).

The baby's name (if given) and sex.

The cause of death (written on the medical certificate).

The parents' full names, occupations (if any), usual address(es) and places of birth. Parents will also be asked other confidential questions for statistical purposes such as their date of birth and date of marriage.

If the parents are not married, and the mother does not want the father's details in the register, her details are sufficient. If they both want his details in the register, contact the registrar for advice about the necessary procedures.

Other information the parents need before they go to the register office

The registrar enters the baby's details and other information in the stillbirth register. Parents may have the baby's forenames entered if they wish, though there is no legal obligation to do this. They may want time to decide the names before they go to the register office.

In **England** and **Wales** the registrar cannot issue a full Certificate of Stillbirth at the time of registration. But he or she should offer to issue a Certificate of Registration of Stillbirth . This is a small piece of thin paper which simply states that the stillbirth has been registered and which can have the baby's forename(s) on it. Parents should be told that if the registrar does not offer to issue a Certificate of Registration of Stillbirth, they can ask for one. It is not possible to get a Certificate of Registration of Stillbirth later.

If parents would also like a certified copy of the full entry in the stillbirth register (a Certificate of Stillbirth), the registrar can arrange to get one for them. This will take about a week. A small fee is payable. Parents should be told before they go to the register office that they can ask the registrar to arrange this, if it is not offered .

If parents did not get a Certificate of Stillbirth at the time of registration, or if they want more copies, they can usually get one by contacting either the register office where they registered the stillbirth (within about three months of registration), or (at any later date) the General Register Office for England and Wales (see USEFUL ADDRESSES page 79).

The registrar will also give the parents a Certificate for

Burial or Cremation (white certificate). They should give this to their funeral director, or, if the hospital is arranging the funeral, to the hospital administrator dealing with it.

In **Scotland** parents can ask the registrar to arrange to get them a Certificate of Stillbirth . This is a certified copy of the full entry in the stillbirth register and should be ready within about a week. A small fee is payable. Parents should be told before they go to the register office that they can ask the registrar to arrange this .

If parents have not asked for a Certificate of Stillbirth at the time of registration, or if they want more copies, they can usually get one by contacting either the register office where they registered the stillbirth (within about three months of registration), or (at any later date) the General Register Office for Scotland (see USEFUL ADDRESSES page 79).

The registrar will also give the parents a Certificate of Registration of Stillbirth. They should give this to their funeral director, or, if the hospital is arranging the funeral, to the hospital administrator dealing with it.

In **Northern Ireland** the registrar will offer parents a copy of the Certificate of Stillbirth when they register the stillbirth. This is an exact copy of the entry in the stillbirth register. A small fee is payable. Additional copies can be got at a later date. Contact the registrar or write to the General Register Office for Northern Ireland (see USEFUL ADDRESSES page 79).

The registrar will also give the parents a form to permit the disposal of the body. They should give this to their funeral director, or, if the hospital is arranging the funeral, to the hospital administrator dealing with it.

Registering a neonatal death

All deaths must normally be registered within five days (eight days in **Scotland**). If it is necessary to go beyond the time limit, contact the registrar as soon as possible.

Both the death and the birth must be registered even if the baby only lived for a few minutes. If the birth has not already been registered, it can be registered at the same time as the death (see below).   See page 53 for coroner's / procurator fiscal's cases.

People who can register a neonatal death

The registrar will normally expect the baby's mother or father to register the death. If this is not possible contact the registrar for advice. If the parents wish to register the baby's birth at the same time and are not married, contact the registrar for advice about the necessary procedures.

Information the registrar will need

The date and place of the baby's death (and the baby's age if he or she lived less than 24 hours).

The cause of death (written on the medical certificate).

The date and place of the baby's birth.

The baby's full name.

The parents' full names, occupations (if any), and home address(es).

If the parents are not married, and the mother does not want the father's details in the register, her details are sufficient. If they both want his details in the register, contact the registrar for advice about the necessary procedures, especially if they intend to register the birth at the same time (see opp.)

Other information the parents need before they go to the register office

The baby's forename(s) can be only entered in the register of deaths at the time of registration. They cannot be entered at a later date. *If the parents have not yet decided on a name, they may want time to think before they go to the register office.*

The registrar will offer the parents certified copies of the baby's entry in the death register, usually known as a Death Certificate. A small fee is payable. Parents can get more copies at a later date by writing to the registrar of the district where the death was registered. If necessary, he or she will refer them to the current holder of the register.

● The registrar will give the parents a Certificate of Burial or Cremation (green form). They should give this to the funeral director or, if the hospital is arranging the funeral, to the hospital administrator dealing with it.

Registering the birth and the death at the same time

● By law, all live births must be registered within six weeks (21 days in Scotland). If the parents have not already registered the baby's birth, they can do this when they register the death. If the parents are not married the father can still register the birth provided the mother has made a statutory declaration stating that he is the baby's father. Contact the registrar for advice about the necessary procedures.

● The baby's forename(s) can be entered on the Birth Certificate.

● If the baby was born in a different registration district from the one in which he or she died, the parents can register the birth 'by declaration' when they register the death. They do not have to register the birth separately. The registrar will send a Declaration of Birth to the registrar of the district in which the baby was born. The latter will send the parents a copy of the baby's Birth Certificate.

● In Scotland and Northern Ireland the birth can be registered either in the district where the baby was born, or in the district where the baby died, or in the district where the mother (or the parents, if married) usually live (providing this is in Scotland or Northern Ireland respectively).

● Parents can get more copies of their baby's Birth Certificate at a later date by writing to the registrar of the district where the birth was registered. If necessary, he or she will refer them to the current holder of the register. A small fee is payable.

● Parents who did not register their baby's forename(s) when they registered the birth may be able to have the name(s) entered up to one year later (two years in Scotland and Northern Ireland). (This is not possible on Death Certificates or for stillbirths.) Parents should contact a registrar for advice.

Registration in coroner's / procurator fiscal's cases

If there are any suspicious circumstances or uncertainties surrounding the cause of death, the doctor or the registrar must report the case to a coroner. In Scotland, the same duties are carried out by a procurator fiscal.

If the coroner takes the case, the doctor does not always give the parents a medical certificate. He or she should tell the parents that the case has been reported, explain why, and outline what is likely to happen next. The doctor should also give the parents the telephone number and address of the coroner's office and encourage them to contact the office.

Unless there is to be an inquest, the coroner will normally send a form to the registrar who will then register the death. The registrar will let the parents know when he or she has received this. Sometimes the coroner will give the form to the parents to take to the registrar.

If there is an inquest, the coroner often opens it and adjourns it as soon as possible (usually within a few days) so that a Burial Order or Cremation Form can be issued. This enables the parents to go ahead with the burial or cremation. Once the inquest is over, the coroner usually sends a certificate to the registrar who then registers the death. The parents can write to the registrar for copies of the baby's Death Certificate as described above. (In the case of a neonatal death the parents must register the birth in the usual way).

Note: The rules affecting the registration of deaths and stillbirths may change when an opportunity arises to legislate on the proposals in the white paper 'Registration: proposals for change'.

Local addresses for registration

Parents should be told the address and hours of opening of the register office. This information should also be written down for them and they should be given a clear detailed map of how to get there.

Registrar's name

Register office address

Telephone number

Hours of opening

Days and times the registrar is at the hospital

Other information

Coroner's / Procurator fiscal's name

Coroner's / Procurator fiscal's office address

Telephone number

Office hours

Other information

Other important information or contacts

CARE AND SUPPORT AT HOME

We received an enormous amount of care and support from the hospital staff both during my stay in hospital and afterwards. When I returned home, my community midwives, health visitor and GP gave us equally good care, support and gentle encouragement to rebuild our lives. What we received from all directions, and was so necessary, was the understanding, time and space to voice our thoughts and ask our endless questions.

(Lynn, whose baby lived for 10 hours 35 minutes)

Many parents who have experienced a miscarriage, stillbirth or neonatal death need care and support from professionals in the community both in the immediate days and weeks after the loss of their baby, and over the following months and years.

Immediate needs

For many parents, going home after the death of their baby or the loss of their pregnancy and having to face the outside world again is painful and hard. It is important that parents do not feel unsupported or rejected by professionals at this time. They may also need practical help and advice.

In the early weeks at home -

- parents will need to talk with professionals about their experience, both separately and together, and may need to ask questions about what happened so that they understand it better

- they may need advice on how to deal with the reactions and questions of other family members (for example, other children, grandparents, a pregnant sister-in-law), and of friends and neighbours

- they may need help in understanding the information they have been given by hospital staff

- they may need advice and help with registering the death or stillbirth (see pages 50-53)

- they may need help in making decisions about and arranging a funeral for their baby (see FUNERALS, BURIALS, CREMATION page 61)

- they may need help and advice on claiming any benefit payments due to them

- women may need help in dealing with physical symptoms such as lactation, stitches, pain, etc. See also HOSPITAL CARE: FOLLOW UP, page 37, for information about the postnatal appointment.

- parents may need to know about local or national voluntary bodies whom they can contact for support and advice (see page 58)

- they may need to talk about the timing of another pregnancy, their chances of having a live healthy baby, and how they can reduce or manage any risks (see page 31)

- they may need to discuss coping with or returning to work.

- they may need help in preparing the questions they want to ask when they see their consultant or GP to discuss the post mortem results (see page 48) or for a follow-up visit

- they may need advice on contraception (see page 31).

Long term support

Over the following months and years parents will continue to grieve for their baby. Many parents will need and value the support of professional staff in going over and validating their memories, and in helping them understand and accept their feelings. Professionals who work in the community will already be aware of the processes of grieving and of the importance of providing opportunities for bereaved people to talk through their experiences and feelings. Professional support given now may help prevent more serious problems later. Professionals working with bereaved parents also need to be aware of the particular difficulties and needs of parents after a miscarriage, a stillbirth or a neonatal death.

Mourning is likely to be especially hard when birth and death are intertwined. It is also more difficult to grieve when there are few if any memories of the baby who has died or when there is nothing tangible to mourn. Parents often need to create and repeat their memories, and to talk through the experience again and again, until it becomes firm in their minds.

Many parents who have lost a baby or whose pregnancy has ended experience grief and distress for several years. This may be the first close bereavement in their lives and they may be unprepared for the pain and sadness to last so long or to keep returning with such strength as time passes. They may worry that they are reacting abnormally.

Friends and relatives often avoid bereaved parents, or are unable or unwilling to listen to them, especially after the first few weeks. If friends and relatives did not know of the pregnancy, the parents' loss may be private and hard to share and their grief may seem in some way unacceptable. Bereaved parents may feel isolated and shut in with their feelings. Skilled community professionals, and parents who have been through a similar experience, are often the only people to whom they feel able to talk freely, especially some months and years after the loss.

Most parents feel a strong need to understand why their baby died or their pregnancy failed. In some cases parents will not have understood or taken in the explanation they were given by the staff in the hospital. They will need further clear and detailed explanation, and opportunities for discussion. If there is thought to have been a hereditary element, they may need help with getting genetic counselling and in understanding and thinking about the implications for future pregnancies. If there are worries that there is a specific medical problem which will recur, they may need to get further help. (For more about giving information see page 9.)

In many cases no satisfying explanation can be found for the death of the baby or the loss of the pregnancy. This can be particularly difficult for parents. They may need help in accepting the absence of a known cause and in believing that they did not somehow cause their baby's death.

The emotions of bereaved parents are likely to fluctuate a good deal. Many events can trigger renewed grieving, for example, the anniversary of the baby's conception, the date on which a baby should have been born, anniversaries of the baby's birth and death, the time at which the baby should have started nursery school or school, and so on. Parents are not always aware of what is causing their sadness at these 'hidden' anniversaries. Traditionally happy family occasions such as summer holidays, and Christmas, or equivalent festivals for members of other faiths, may rekindle grief.

The loss of one twin may be particularly difficult since parents need both to focus on and grieve for the baby who died, and to develop a relationship with the baby who has lived. Other people often encourage them to ignore their loss and to be happy with the baby they still have, but to the parents both babies are equally valuable, and it is very important that the dead baby should be recognised and mourned in his or her own right and as one of twins. Many parents also feel some resentment at the live twin who they may feel has survived at the expense of the twin who died. It may help them to know that this feeling is not unusual and that they do not need to feel ashamed of it.

Other people's pregnancies and new babies can be difficult and distressing for bereaved parents, who often feel shocked at the strength of their jealousy and anger.

Family relationships People mourn at different rates and show their grief in different ways. For some people, their grieving may be also exacerbated and complicated by previous bereavements and losses. Grieving partners may find it difficult to listen sympathetically to each other, since both are in urgent need of support and comfort.

● All members of the family may be affected by the baby's death. For example, other children may be upset and frightened, both by the death itself and by their parents' grief and other reactions. They are very likely to show their unhappiness by changes in behaviour and by becoming more demanding. This can add to parents' worry and distress. Parents may also find it hard to meet the needs of the other children in the family at a time when they need so much care themselves.

● Children vary in their emotional awareness, but the depth of understanding of even comparatively young children should not be underestimated. Giving children an honest account of what has happened can help to reduce possible fears and guilt. Even an early miscarriage may have an impact on a child and require an explanation. Some children also worry that in some way they caused the loss of the baby or that they too will die.

● Grandparents are often severely affected by the death of a baby. They have lost a grandchild and must also watch their own child suffering the pain of bereavement. If the grandparents themselves had a miscarriage, stillbirth or neonatal death in their childbearing years, this new loss may reawaken strong feelings of grief, anger and distress. If there are difficulties in the relationships with parents and in-laws, these can become worse after the death of a baby.

● If there were problems and conflicts in relationships within the family before the baby died, these may increase.

● **The next pregnancy** The timing of another pregnancy, the risks involved, and the chances of a live healthy baby are urgent concerns for many parents. They need information and also opportunities to talk and ask questions, so that they can make an informed decision. They need to be aware that if the new baby is conceived fairly quickly, he or she is likely to be born around the first anniversary of the baby who died and this can be very hard. An early pregnancy may sometimes prevent the full course of grieving: suppressed grief may recur at the birth of the new baby and may be more difficult to deal with.

● The next pregnancy can give rise to complicated and difficult emotions. Parents are naturally likely to be particularly anxious and to need sympathetic support and information as it progresses. It may be hard not to see the expected baby as in some ways a replacement for the one who died.

● If the pregnancy results in a live healthy baby, parents are often suprised and confused by the strength of the renewed grief they may feel for the baby who died, and by the mixed feelings they may have for the new baby. Relatives and friends may find these reactions hard to understand and upsetting.

Professional roles

Professionals can have an important role to play when a pregnancy has failed or a baby has died.

If one person in the professional team already has a good relationship with the parents, it is often most appropriate for him or her to visit first. Coordination of care is then vital. It is useful if all the community professionals in touch with a bereaved family meet to discuss together the needs of family members and how these can be met. In the long term, parents often find it helpful if they know that there is one key professional who will keep in regular touch with them and whom they can contact to ask for a visit or just when they need to talk.

Since care needs to be provided for both parents it may be necessary to arrange some visits in the evenings and at weekends.

Community midwives have a statutory responsibility to visit at home mothers of all babies born alive at any gestation, and mothers of all babies stillborn after 28 weeks gestation. They must visit up to at least 10 days after the birth and can continue to visit up to 28 days. In some districts all women whose babies have died at any gestation are offered a visit from a community midwife.

In most places **health visitors** carry out at least one postnatal visit to each mother at home with her new baby. This should also be done wherever possible for those mothers whose babies have died after birth or were born dead. At this visit, the health visitor can assess whether further visits would be helpful and can encourage parents who wish to make contact with local self help groups. In some areas the hospital informs the health visitor when a woman miscarries at any gestation so that she can be offered a follow-up visit.

Health visitors and community midwives may also be able to help set up local self-help groups with women who have experienced a miscarriage, stillbirth or neonatal death. They can advise and support as necessary, working closely with local voluntary organisations where these exist.

The **GP** may have an important role in explaining and discussing the post mortem / investigation report and its implications with the parents. He or she may also need to refer parents for genetic counselling, to give them contraceptive advice, to support them through the next pregnancy, and, where necessary, to refer them for special counselling and support.

In areas with a high turnover of other community professionals, the GP may also be extremely important as the one professional in touch with and supporting bereaved parents over many years and as a source of information about their past and present situation for newly arrived community staff.

The community midwife will be informed of all spontaneous abortions and terminations for medical reasons at the discretion of the gynaecology ward staff who will elicit the feelings of the parents. The community midwife will visit the woman on the day following discharge and then as necessary.

(Grimsby Health Authority)

I think the person who helped me most is my health visitor. She came every week for an hour to give me a chance to talk. That time was for me to pour out my grief to someone who didn't object to my tears or tell me what I should or should not do.

(Hayriye, whose baby lived for 3 months)

In some areas there are also other professionals who have a special role with bereaved parents, for example, a bereavement counsellor, a chaplain with special responsibility for maternity care, a social worker, a neonatal or gynaecological liaison sister, a family care sister. They need to work closely with other professionals in the community to avoid duplication and ensure that care is coordinated. They may also have an important role in advising and supporting community professionals in their work with bereaved parents.

Communication between the hospital and the community

Good communication between hospital and community staff is essential to ensure both that parents receive the support they need as soon as they go home, and that they are not caused unnecessary distress because the appropriate community staff have not been told of their loss. (For more information, see 'Communication with community staff', page 26.)

Information for parents

Parents need to know what professional and voluntary support is available to them in the community and how they can get it. They need verbal explanations, backed up by written information. (For more information see HOSPITAL CARE: POSTNATAL CARE page 32.)

Voluntary support

Many parents get invaluable support from talking to other parents who have been through a similar experience. Sharing thoughts and feelings with other bereaved parents can provide a different kind of support from that given by professionals. Professionals need to know about local and national voluntary groups and schemes, what

**SANDS
befrienders are
here to listen
when others can
listen no more.
Befrienders are
not trained
counsellors, but
they can give
grieving parents
what they most
need: acceptance
of their loss and a
listener who
understands that
to talk about the
baby you have
lost is both
healthy and
necessary.**

(Mallinson G, 'When a
baby dies', Nursing
Times, 1 March 1989,
Vol 85, No 9, 31-4)

they offer, and how to contact them.

All bereaved parents should be offered information about relevant groups and given the names of local group contacts or befrienders where possible. Professionals should offer to make the first contact with the group if the parents wish. It is important that voluntary and professional support are seen as complementary, and that professionals do not withdraw their support once parents have developed local contacts.

National addresses of voluntary organisations that offer support and information for bereaved parents are given in USEFUL ADDRESSES page 78.

A policy for care in the community

Community professionals in each area need to develop a clear policy in order to ensure that all parents who have had a miscarriage, stillbirth or neonatal death can get the care and support they need. This should include -

- criteria for providing care

- the types of care and support that can be offered to bereaved parents locally and how they can get access to them

- an outline of the separate and shared roles of the different professionals working with bereaved parents

- a description of how effective communication and coordination will be achieved between professionals in the community, and between hospital and community professionals

- details of relevant local voluntary organisations and a policy for collaboration with them in providing support for bereaved parents

- an outline of the day-to-day support and supervision to be provided for community professionals working with bereaved families and also how they can get access to specialist counselling and support whenever necessary

A clear policy will help avoid duplication of effort and ensure that resources are directed where they are most needed.

Local information: voluntary organisations

(see also page 78)

Local MA contact

Address

Tel No

Local SANDS contact

Address

Tel No

Local TAMBA contact

Address

Tel No

Local BLISSLINK contact

Address

Tel No

Local NIPPERS contact

Address

Tel No

Local SATFA contact

Address

Tel No

Local NCT contact

Address

Tel No

Local FSID/SCDT contact

Address

Tel No

Other useful contacts

FUNERALS, BURIALS, CREMATION

I had carried that child inside of me for 7 months, loved her from the moment she existed, and I wanted to know where and how she had been laid to rest. It helps me to know where she is, to go and take flowers and be as close to her as I can.

(Lyn, whose baby was stillborn)

* At the time of publication the age of viability is legally defined as 28 weeks gestation. It is expected that this will be lowered.

For many parents the death of their baby is their first experience of a death in the family. They may have no knowledge of the arrangements that have to be made nor of the wide range of choices open to them. It is also very hard for parents to cope with arrangements to do with death when they have so recently been planning their baby's future.

Parents whose baby has died need help and support so that they can make the decisions that are right for them. Later it will be very important to have positive memories of what they did (or what was done) for their baby.

What parents need to decide

In the days and weeks after the death of their baby, parents need to decide -

- what kind of funeral they want

- who will organise and pay for the funeral

- whether their baby should be buried or cremated.

Formal burial or cremation is legally required for all babies who are stillborn or die after birth. However, it is important not to assume that parents of those babies who are born dead before the legal age of viability* will not also want a formal burial or cremation for their baby. See page 67 for more information on the options for these babies and also MEMORIALS page 73.

Time to decide

Parents should not be put under unnecessary pressure to make decisions about their baby's funeral in a hurry (but see box). Many parents initially find the idea of involving themselves in their baby's funeral shocking and distressing, but given time and encouragement, begin to appreciate the opportunity to do so, and later are glad that they did. It can also take time to feel clear about how best to honour and mourn a lost baby, and opportunities missed now can never be made up. Occasionally it may be necessary to wait for some weeks until a mother comes out of hospital.

Hospital arrangements for the storage of babies' bodies should give parents enough time to make their decisions. Parents should be told that their baby's body will be kept safely. They should also be told if there is a time limit after which their baby's body cannot be kept. (See 'Storage of babies' bodies', page 25.)

As far as possible, both parents should be involved in all discussions about the funeral.

For parents of some religious faiths it is important that the funeral should take place as soon as possible, usually within 24 hours. This may be true for Orthodox Jews, Muslims, Hindus and Sikhs and also for some Christian groups. These parents may need the help of hospital staff to get the necessary certification completed urgently (see also page 42).

The value of a funeral

A funeral can be religious or non-religious. Even a religious ceremony can take many different forms. Parents should be encouraged to organise whatever ceremony will meet their own needs. Hospital chaplains can often help parents with widely differing wishes find a form of ceremony that suits them.

For many parents, arranging or participating in some kind of ceremony, no matter how simple or private, helps to give reality and expression to their loss. A ceremony can also play a very important part in making the baby's existence real for family and friends, and gives them a formal opportunity to express their sympathy and support.

In some cases, parents may be able to choose between organising a funeral themselves and allowing the hospital to organise and pay for it. For more about the different options see below.

Professional support and guidance

In order to make these difficult decisions, parents need information, guidance and support. Local regulations regarding burials and cremations vary tremendously, and the bereavement officer or other professional who discusses the options with parents needs to be familiar with the regulations and possibilities in his or her area. He or she needs to be well informed about -

- what *must* be done and what *can* be done locally for babies miscarried or born dead at all gestations, and for babies who died shortly after birth

- arrangements in the case of a hospital funeral (see Opposite) and what options the parents have to enhance the funeral (see pages 66-67).

- what, in general terms, is involved if parents organise the funeral themselves and what options they have (see pages 63-67).

Useful sources of information may include local funeral directors, clergy, and cemetery and crematorium authorities.

Certification for a funeral

The funeral director will need the certificate issued by the registrar (white in the case of a stillborn baby, green in the case of a neonatal death) in order to go ahead with the funeral. Additional medical certificates will be needed if a stillborn baby or a baby who died shortly after death is to be cremated (see pages 48-49 for details). The parents will also need to give their written consent.

There is no registrar's certificate nor cremation form for a baby born dead before the legal age of viability since the death is not registered. In this case the doctor or midwife who attended the delivery should issue a certificate or letter for the funeral director (see page 48 for more about this).

A funeral arranged by the hospital

In the case of a stillborn baby, the hospital should always offer to arrange and pay for a funeral if the parents would find this helpful (see *Funerals for Stillborn Babies* DHSS 1975, and DHSS circulars DS211/75 and HN(76)18, updated in HN(85)31. Some hospitals also offer to arrange and pay for the funerals of babies who were born dead before the legal age of viability or who died a few days or weeks after birth.

If the parents choose, the hospital may take full responsibility for arranging the funeral. The parents then need only decide whether they want their baby buried or cremated (see page 64). They are not obliged to attend the funeral but can if they wish.

However, for many parents there are emotional risks in letting the hospital take responsibility for the funeral. They can too easily lose control over, and contact with, what happens to their baby. Even those parents who feel that they cannot bear to be involved at the time, may later bitterly regret their decision.

To prevent such regrets, it is important that even when parents ask the hospital to arrange and pay for their baby's funeral, they are still encouraged and enabled to take part in planning the funeral and to attend. The parents should be given the name of the funeral director with whom the hospital has a contract. They should be encouraged to contact the funeral director to discuss the basic form of funeral they would like and decide on any extras they wish to pay for themselves. Some parents may initially prefer a member of the hospital or community staff to liaise with the funeral director for them but it is important that they are given every opportunity to make decisions themselves and to become involved.

If a family already has a funeral director, some hospitals will pay the basic contract fee to him or her provided the funeral director meets at least the minimum standards laid down in the hospital contract (see below).

Hospitals may also sometimes need to use a specialist funeral director who is experienced in, for example, Jewish or Muslim funerals, and who has links with appropriate cemeteries.

Parents whose baby's funeral is arranged by the hospital should always be told the time and place of the funeral and invited to attend, accompanied by a member of staff from the hospital or the community if they wish. If they decide not to attend and the baby is buried, the funeral director should make sure that they are informed sensitively where the grave is and the number of the plot.

If the parents would like a religious funeral service, the hospital chaplain or the funeral director should put them in touch with the appropriate minister if necessary, so that they can discuss the form of service.

The hospital contract

In its contract with a local funeral director the hospital should state clearly its requirements for funerals for babies. The contract should also lay down that parents must be able to discuss the funeral with the funeral director beforehand, to participate as much as they wish, and to enhance the funeral by paying for additional features not included in the contract. These could include, for example, a second car to take other family members to the funeral, flowers, a different type of coffin (some parents do not like the traditional white coffin), and having the baby at home before the funeral.

It is very important that parents who choose a hospital funeral do not feel that they are giving their baby a 'cheap' and therefore inferior option. The hospital must ensure that the standard of a hospital funeral is at least as good as that of a simple private funeral and parents must be assured that this is so.

The administrator or midwife responsible should attend hospital funerals regularly to monitor the standard of provision and ensure that it is acceptable.

A revised specimen contract between a hospital and a funeral director is set out on pages 71 and 72. This has been drawn up by representatives of the Association of National Health Service Supplies Officers and the British Institute of Funeral Directors. It sets out the *minimum* acceptable standard which SANDS recommends for a baby's funeral. Hospitals should only consider those tenders that meet their agreed standards. These are unlikely to be the cheapest.

Note: The term 'contract funeral' sounds uncaring to lay ears and should not normally be used when talking to parents or relatives.

A funeral arranged by the parents

If parents are organising the funeral themselves, it is still important that a well-informed hospital or community professional is available to discuss the possibilities with them, and to give support.

Parents may need reassurance that a private funeral need not be difficult to arrange or expensive. It may require only one or two visits or telephone calls to a local funeral director to discuss what is wanted. Sometimes another member of the family or a close friend whom the parents trust to consult them fully and follow their wishes may be prepared to take on the practical arrangements.

Some funeral directors charge very little or even nothing for private funerals of stillborn or very young babies, though parents have to pay extra for any additional features. Parents also have to pay any local charges for burial or cremation (see page 66).

If the parents are organising the funeral themselves, the hospital should give them a list of local funeral directors. This should also indicate members of the British Institute of Funeral Directors and/or of the National Association of Funeral Directors. Parents should be told that they are free to go to any funeral director, and that they can discuss costs and find out what different funeral directors would provide without making any commitment.

Funeral directors can be very helpful and parents should be encouraged to contact them as soon as they feel able, to discuss what they want. The funeral director should talk through with the parents what is possible and what they might like, guiding them through the procedures and making suggestions as appropriate. The funeral director should do his or her best to ensure that the parents are able to create the best possible funeral for their baby. Some parents may prefer a member of the hospital or community staff to liaise with the funeral director for them but it is important that they are still given every opportunity to make decisions themselves and to become involved.

The parents may also like to get in touch with their local SANDS or other bereavement support group (see page 60) to find out what can be done locally and to get personal recommendations of local funeral directors.

The parents will need to decide whether they want their baby buried or cremated (see opposite). If the parents want a religious funeral service the funeral director or hospital chaplain should offer to contact a minister for them if necessary.

Deciding on burial or cremation

In order to decide whether to have their baby's body buried or cremated, parents need to know what is involved in either choice and what facilities are available locally. In some cases there are inflexible local regulations which affect parents' options. Local funeral directors will be well informed about these, but it is useful for the professionals who are supporting parents to have a general understanding of the local situation.

Some religions permit only cremation, though burial may sometimes be preferred for a very young baby. Some religions permit only burial.

Cremation

Parents should be told if there will be no cremated remains (ashes). This is because the soft bones of very small babies are usually destroyed by the high temperatures of the cremation process. A few crematoria can now provide the ashes of very small babies.

Parents may be able to put up a small memorial plaque or stone if they wish in the crematorium grounds. There may be several options for them to choose from. They may wish to visit the crematorium grounds in advance to see what is possible. It may also be possible to put up a memorial plaque in a local churchyard.

In some crematoria there is a special garden where the ashes (if any) of very young babies can be scattered. Sometimes parents can have their baby's name inscribed on a special memorial stone there. Alternatively, if there are ashes, parents may be able to bury them in a local churchyard or municipal cemetery, possibly with a plaque. This may be closer to their home and easier for them to visit. Some parents may prefer to scatter any ashes in a place with a special meaning to them.

All crematoria have books of remembrance in which parents can enter their baby's name and an inscription (see page 73).

A memorial plot has been purchased at the crematorium and this is planted with shrubs etc where parents can visit whenever they wish.

(Royal Devon and Exeter Hospital, Heavitree)

Burial

If parents are considering burial, they may find it helpful to visit the cemetery to see where their baby would be buried. They also need to know whether the cemetery regulations will allow them to bury their baby in a way that they find acceptable.

In some municipal cemeteries, all babies, whether given a hospital or private funeral, are buried in separate graves. In other places, stillborn and very young babies (especially those who are given hospital contract funerals) can only be buried in a grave shared with a number of other babies, each in his or her own coffin. The number of babies in a grave varies. In 1986, SANDS, in their publication, *After Stillbirth* , recommended that no more than ten babies should be buried in one grave, and that these graves should be located in a special children's area of the cemetery with a general memorial stone and a book of remembrance for individual entries. In a few places, babies are still buried in large general graves with a number of adults and other babies.

Some hospitals have bought a special plot in a nearby cemetery where babies of all gestations and ages can be buried. There is usually a shared memorial stone on which parents can sometimes have the details of their baby entered. In some places parents can put up individual stones.

Some parents may prefer to have their baby buried in a nearby or familiar churchyard. Whether this is possible will depend on the church regulations. Muslim and Jewish parents may wish their baby to be buried in a special cemetery reserved for members of their faith.

If possible, professionals advising parents should visit local cemeteries so that they can describe them to parents and also warn parents in advance of things that they may find distressing.

A shared grave Some parents find it comforting to know that their baby will be buried in a grave with other babies. Others find the idea of a shared grave upsetting. It is

There are no common graves into which more than one child is buried...Marked graves are allowed - even encouraged.

(Rev Tony Porter, Hospital chaplain, Maidstone Hospital)

Burial of babies born dead before the legal age of viability

Some municipal cemeteries do not permit the burial of these babies. However, if there is a local churchyard with space, the incumbent may allow the baby to be buried there. Some incumbents do not allow plaques for these babies.

---

important that parents do not find out that their baby is in a shared grave when it is too late for them to consider alternatives. (Once closed, a shared grave cannot be reopened unless all the families involved and the Home Office give their consent. This is not normally feasible.)

Parents should be told in advance if their baby is likely to be buried in a shared grave, how many babies or coffins there will be in the grave, and how long it is likely to be before the grave is closed and the ground properly reinstated.

Some cemeteries do not permit headstones of any kind, individual or shared, on a shared grave. Others do, but lay down the type and size of headstone that is permitted. Where a headstone is not permitted, there is sometimes a shared memorial stone nearby and it may be possible to have the baby's name and dates of birth and death engraved on this. There may also be a book of remembrance at the cemetery in which parents can have their baby's name entered, with an inscription if they choose. Rules in some cemeteries forbid any flowers on a shared grave.

In many places, the regulations governing shared graves are still not as parents would like them to be. It is most important that parents whose baby may be buried in a shared grave are told in advance what is and is not permitted locally so that they do not discover too late that they cannot bury or commemorate their baby in the way that they planned.

Note: the term 'common grave' has unpleasant associations for many parents, and even more for many grandparents, and should be avoided.

A private plot Parents who buy a private burial plot may wish to mark their baby's grave with a headstone. All cemeteries have regulations affecting the size and type of headstone that can be put up and when this can be done. Parents need to know about these in advance.

For advice on gravestones and memorials, parents can

The National Association
of Master Masons,
Crown Buildings,
High Street,
Aylesbury,
Bucks HP20 1SL
(0296 434 750)

The Memorial Advisory
Bureau,
139 Kensington High
Street,
London W8 6SX
(071 937 0052)

contact a local funeral director or monumental mason, the National Association of Master Masons, or the Memorial Advisory Bureau (addresses opposite). Their local SANDS or other bereavement support group may also be able to give advice.

Some families already have a grave plot, with another member of the family buried in it. They can normally bury the baby there, provided they have the owner's written authority. There will be a fee for reopening the grave and for the burial, and also for adding an inscription to the headstone if parents wish.

The cost of a funeral

For many parents the cost of the different options will be a factor in their decision.

● If the hospital arranges and pays for the funeral (see page 62), this will include the cost of burial (often in a shared grave) or cremation. Parents may decide whether they wish to pay for any enhancements to the funeral, for a headstone, or for any other additions.

● For a private funeral for a baby, most funeral directors charge only a nominal fee. However, parents still have to pay the full costs charged by the crematorium or cemetery authorities, and any other costs, such as fees for a church service, if wanted.

● For a cremation, costs include the crematorium fees and, if the parents wish, the cost of a memorial plaque or some other form of memorial.

● For a burial, the cost of buying a private plot in a municipal cemetery can be very high. In some cemeteries it is possible to buy a smaller child's plot which is less expensive. Alternatively it may be possible to buy a place in a shared grave. A few families may already have a family plot (see above). There will be a charge for digging or reopening the grave. Parents may also wish to buy a headstone for their baby's grave if this is permitted. Burial in

a churchyard, if local church regulations permit, is far less expensive, though there will still be additional fees, for example, for digging the grave.

It is important that the professional who is supporting the parents knows the kinds of sums that the different choices will involve, and is also able to reassure parents that the amount of money they spend on their baby's funeral is in no way a measure of their love for their baby or of their grief at his or her death.

Help from the state   Parents who receive Income Support, Family Credit or Housing Benefit may be able (depending on the level of any savings) to get a lump sum tax-free payment towards funeral costs. This covers the cost of a simple funeral and cemetery or cremation fees. Parents can apply to the Social Fund on Claim Form SF200 (available from the local social security office or the registrar of births and deaths) and will need to supply an estimate or bill from the funeral director. They must claim within three months of the funeral. The hospital social worker or the bereavement officer can advise parents on how to claim.

Hospital Trustees' Funds   Some hospitals make a contribution out of Trustees' Funds towards funeral costs for parents who are in financial difficulties and are not eligible for a Social Fund payment.

If the baby was delivered or transferred to a unit distant from the parents' home, the hospital will arrange for the body to be transported back to the home area for the funeral free of charge.

Making the most of the funeral

Parents whose babies never lived outside the womb, or who died shortly after birth, can find it particularly difficult to grieve for someone whom they may feel they never got the chance to know properly and of whom they have few or no memories. Creating special memories around the baby can be very important, both now and for later. It is important to make the most of the opportunities the funeral ceremony offers for this, and to make it as individual as possible to those parents and their baby.

For example, parents may gain comfort from such things as -

- their baby being dressed in his or her own clothes in the coffin

- placing one or two special things in the coffin, for example, a family photograph, a letter or poem to the baby, drawings or paintings by siblings, a soft toy such as a teddy bear, something they had bought specially for the baby, a rose, or something else of special value and significance to them. (Crematorium safety rules do not allow anything except paper and clothing to be cremated with a body. If the baby is to be cremated, anything else placed in the coffin will be removed by the funeral director before it is finally closed and will be given back to the parents.)

- having the baby at home the night before the funeral, with the lid of the coffin left open if the parents wish

- taking the coffin to the funeral with them in the funeral director's limousine or in their own car

- carrying the coffin from the car to the chapel and then to the grave or the crematorium

- choosing special readings, songs or hymns for the funeral
- making the funeral service special and individual to that baby and that family in any way they can think of.

Parents may need help and support in thinking about what they can do to ensure that their baby's funeral is right for them. See also **MEMORIALS** page 73.

Babies born dead before the legal age of viability: possible arrangements

There is no legal requirement to bury or cremate a baby born dead before the legal age of viability. However, since the acceptance of the Polkinghorne Report '*Review of the Guidance on the Research Use of Fetuses and Fetal Material*' (HMSO 1989) by the Department of Health, all parents must be asked how their baby's body should be disposed of.

'*... we would like to record our belief that on general ethical grounds of respect, all mothers .... should be given the opportunity clearly to express their wishes about the eventual disposal of the dead fetus, and that these wishes should, wherever possible, be respected*' (6.12)

Many parents of babies born dead before the legal age of viability will want to hold a funeral or some other kind of religious or non-religious ceremony for their baby as described in the previous pages. Some parents may not think spontaneously of having a funeral or other ceremony but will welcome the idea if it is suggested to them. Others will not want to have any kind of ceremony for themselves, but will, nonetheless, find it important that their baby's body is treated with care and dignity.

It is important that professionals do not assume that parents of these babies will not want a funeral or other recognition of their baby simply because of the timing of their loss. All parents should be given information and guidance to help them think through what they want and should be encouraged to organise whatever they feel is most appropriate. Parents who want a religious ceremony may like to go to their own vicar, priest, rabbi or other minister or may prefer to ask the hospital chaplain to find a form of service that meets their needs.

The body of a baby born before the legal age of viability should not be disposed of until the parents have decided what they would like to do.

If a fetus is identified it is ... cremated at the public crematorium with a service conducted by the chaplain ... Midwives, doctors and administrators attend as do mortuary staff and pathologists. Relatives and friends are invited personally but a public notice is placed in the local paper announcing the time and the place of the service; a wreath is given by the Health Board and usually joined by sprays and wreaths from the relatives. Should parents not wish this, they can either arrange a private cremation or burial, or a hospital burial.

(Aberdeen Maternity Hospital)

Respectful storage and disposal

If parents of a baby born dead before the legal age of viability decide not to hold a funeral, they may need to know what will happen to their baby's body. Disposal by the hospital must be respectful and dignified.

Although in most hospitals the normal method of disposal of the bodies of these babies will be incineration, some parents will, for religious reasons, be unable to agree to this. In these cases at least, the hospital should make provision for burial. Alternatively, some parents may wish to take their baby's body out of the hospital for burial (see below).

SANDS recommends that -

- all hospitals should have an agreed policy for the respectful disposal of bodies of babies for whom no other arrangement has been made

- all bodies of whatever gestation should be stored individually and decently until disposal

- each body should be identified (see page 25).

It is very important that the hospital's policy on what is done with the bodies of babies born before the legal age of viability for whom no other arrangement has been made should be acceptable to representatives of bereaved parents (eg, local SANDS and Miscarriage Association groups), to representatives of the main local religious communities, and to the staff who will have to explain it and carry it out. In some cases, staff may need training and support in carrying out new policies.

Possible arrangements are:

● In some hospitals, all bodies are incinerated once a month after a short committal service conducted by the hospital chaplain. Parents may be invited to come to a service in the hospital chapel at which their baby's name is read out and they can make an entry in a book of remembrance if they wish. The chaplain attends the incineration.

● Some hospitals organise for all bodies for whom no other arrangement has been made to be taken once a month (or once a fortnight) to the local crematorium. The hospital chaplain conducts a short service before the cremation. Parents are invited to attend the ceremony, the baby's names can be read out during the ceremony if parents wish and they can bring flowers.

● Some hospitals have purchased a special burial area in the local cemetery where the bodies of all babies, born alive or dead, and at whatever gestation, can be buried.

● Some hospitals use a separate incinerator for bodies of babies born dead before the legal age of viability for whom no other arrangements have been made. Even if they decide not to hold a funeral, parents of these babies may still like to organise a service of prayer or blessing. The hospital chaplain can usually help with this if parents wish. (See also MEMORIALS page 73.)

Disposal by the parents

Since babies born dead before the legal age of viability do not by law have to be formally buried or cremated, some parents choose to dispose of their baby's body themselves without involving a funeral director. There is no legal reason why this should not be done. The hospital should support the parents and should provide an appropriate container in which they can take the body or the products of conception. No documentation is legally necessary though the hospital may wish to give the parents a letter or certificate as described on page 48, and a release form for the mortuary.

Fetal remains of any gestation are treated exactly the same as stillbirth. The only paperwork required is a statement from the doctor or midwife attending the delivery, together with a standard Notice of Interment. Interment is recorded in the Burial Register, and individual memorials are allowed.

(The London Borough of Brent, and Norwich City Council)

Local information for hospital staff: funeral directors, cemeteries, crematoria

Where to find the hospital list of local funeral directors

Name of the contract funeral director used by the hospital

Address

Telephone number

Other information

Cemetery used by the hospital

Address

Telephone number

Where to find copies of map and directions

Current practice for hospital funerals

Single graves?

Shared graves -

   babies only?

   adults and babies?

How many in one grave?

How long before ground is reinstated?

General memorial stone for babies in shared graves?

Other important information

Crematorium used by the hospital

Address

Telephone number

Arrangements for individual memorials?

Where to find copies of map and directions

Other important information

Hospital arrangements for disposal of babies born dead before the legal age of viability and products of conception

Other important information

Specimen contract for the funerals of babies born dead before the legal age of viability, stillborn babies and neonates

Notes

When considering a contract for these funerals, authorities are advised to assess carefully what is offered by funeral directors to ensure that the service and facilities provided under a contract arrangement are equivalent to those available for a private funeral.

It is advisable that companies selected to tender should be members of the National Association of Funeral Directors and that funeral directors should be members of the British Institute of Funeral Directors. Both have strict codes of practice and a national impartial procedure for dealing with complaints.

It is considered that a contract should be reviewed every 3 years.

The National Association of Funeral Directors
618 Warwick Road
Solihull
West Midlands
B91 1AA
Telephone 021 711 1343

The British Institute of Funeral Directors
11 Regent Street
Kingswood
Bristol
BS15 2JX
Telephone 0272 614737

Contract for the funeral of a stillborn child, neonate, and non-viable foetus

Period   (3 years)

Specification

1. Supply of coffins - construction

1.1 **Spec. 1 (Minimum)**
The coffin should be a rectangular box constructed of composition board, covered with white fabric on the outside. The lid of the coffin should be fitted with an identification plate fixed with two screws, the inside lined with white satinised PVC and appropriately trimmed. Approximate internal dimensions 22" x 8" x7". Suitable for Burial or Cremation.

1.2 **Spec. 2 (Alternative)**
The coffin should be suitable for burial or cremation to size required. To be constructed of composition board covered with Oak, Elm, Beech or Mahogany wood veneer. The outside to be fitted with four handles and the lid to be secured with four screws and fittings and mounted with an engraved identification plate bearing name, age and date of death of deceased. The inside to be lined in white satinised PVC with pillow and appropriately trimmed. Fittings may be electro-brassed or nickel-plated plastic.

2. Funeral arrangements

2.1 The Funeral Director shall convey the baby from the hospital to the Chapel of Rest and subsequently to the Cemetery or Crematorium as decided using a hearse or estate car for the purpose. If an estate car is used it must be conducive to normal funeral practice.

2.2 The Funeral Director shall attend the funeral whether witnessed or not by relatives and shall ensure that all arrangements are conducted in a dignified respectful manner.

2.3 The Funeral Director shall act upon the instructions of the designated Hospital Officer.

3. Service

Funeral Directors will be required to provide the following facilities:
3.1 To offer the use of the Chapel of Rest (to enable the Body to be removed from the environment of the Hospital Mortuary and for family viewing).

3.2 To arrange with immediate family and/or relatives to attend the funeral at a time to suit mourners wherever possible and to arrange with the Minister of Religion, if requested, to attend and conduct a service.

3.3 To arrange collection and collation of all documentation related to the Funeral.

3.4 To arrange payment of all Fees and disbursements related to the Funeral. (When invoiced to Authority, items to be shown separately.)

3.5 To offer help, guidance and advice to relatives on matters outside the contract sphere, i.e. re flowers, memorials, remembrance book, etc. (These items to be at direct cost to family/relatives.)

4. Supplementary options

The Authority may from time to time request that the following optional extras are provided by the Funeral Director.

4.1 The conveying of the body to the home of the parents.

4.2 A Church Service.

4.3 The re-opening of a Private Grave.

4.4 Book of Remembrance.

4.5 Extra limousine(s) for Mourners.

5. Invoicing for service provided

Each Funeral to be invoiced separately showing clearly the Hospital Order Number.

Schedule of prices

Description of service	Tendered price exc. VAT
1 Coffin as spec. 1 - burial	
cremation	
2 Coffin as spec. 2 - burial	
cremation	
3 Conveying of body from hospital to Chapel of Rest	
4 Provisions of hearse/estate car and bearers	
5 Separate conveyance for mourners	
6 Provision of crucifix for Roman Catholic denomination	
7 Conveying of body to hospital mortuary if necessary	

Special conditions of contract

1. Duration of contract

The contract is to commence on   and continue until   . The contract shall continue in force for the period indicated in the tender documents but shall be subject to termination at the end of three months or at any time thereafter provided one month's notice in writing shall have previously been given by either party.

The termination of the contract as regards any one or more of the said items, shall not preclude either party from subsequently determining the Contract by notice as aforesaid as regards any other of the said items. In the event of any breach on the part of the Contractor of the Standard Conditions of Contract, or summarily, by the Authority, who shall give written notice of such determination to the Contractor, and the Authority shall not be liable to pay any sum by way of compensation or otherwise, to the Contractor and shall be entitled to recover from the Contractor an loss resulting from such determination.

2 Price

Subject to any special provision in the Schedule, the contract price shall be net, all cash and trade discounts being allowed. The amount of any VAT or duty included in the Contract price shall be shown in the Schedule.

3. Price changes

Without prejudice to its rights under Condition No.1, Duration of Contract, the Authority may agree to changes in the Contract Price at the end of the three month or any time thereafter, provided not less that one calendar months notice in writing of proposed changes shall have been given by the Contractor.

The Contractor shall at the request of the Authority, furnish such books, accounts documents and records and such other information as the Authority may reasonably require to verify the changes in costs incurred by the Contractor.

4. Arbitration

All disputes, differences or questions between the parties to the Contract with respect to any matter or thing arising out of, or relating to the Contract other than a matter or thing as to which the decision of the Authority is under the contract to be final and conclusive (and except to the extent to which special provision for arbitration is made elsewhere in the Contract) shall be referred to the arbitration of two persons (one to be appointed by the Authority and one by the Contractor) or their Umpire, in accordance with the provisions of the Arbitration Act 1950.

Contractor

Address

Signed

Designation

Date

Tenders are requested to provide the following information:

1. British institute of Funeral Directors

Name of Member

Membership No.

2. National Association of Funeral Directors

Branch

MEMORIALS

Many parents feel a strong wish to have some kind of lasting memorial to their baby. In the months and years to come, physical reminders of their baby's life, however short, will often be very important. A formal memorial such as a headstone or a plaque in a cemetery or in the crematorium grounds (see pages 64-66) may mark a place that is special to their baby, though the possibility of this depends on local regulations. Many parents will want to create other memorials to their baby and will often be grateful for suggestions from well-informed and experienced professionals. They may also like to contact their local SANDS, Miscarriage Association or other bereavement support group (see page 60) to find out what other parents have done.

Books of remembrance

All crematoria and some cemeteries have a book of remembrance in which parents can have their baby's name and an inscription of their choice entered. The funeral director or the local crematorium or cemetery manager can tell them how to arrange this.

Many neonatal units and labour wards now also have books of remembrance. These are sometimes kept in the hospital chapel. Parents of all babies who died shortly after birth, or who were born dead at any gestational age, should be offered the opportunity to enter their baby's name and an inscription of their choice.

It is important to ensure that the book of remembrance, hospital remembrance and sympathy cards and other similar material do not offend or exclude non-Christian parents.

A service of remembrance for lost babies was held. Over 100 people gathered in the church. We were pleased and very touched to see that they included midwives, families, people alone, young and mature couples, babies, children and several elderly people.

(Sue Howitt, Cheltenham SANDS)

For parents who have lost their baby, a Memorial Book is kept on SCBU. Parents can see the book, write in the book, or request an entry to be made by the staff.

(Royal Devon and Exeter Hospital, (Heavitree))

Memorial ceremonies

Parents who have decided not to arrange or attend a funeral, or who have lost their baby early in pregnancy, may wish to organise or attend a memorial ceremony. This can be held shortly after the death or later. Many parents have found such a ceremony helpful and comforting even many years later.

Parents who want a religious memorial ceremony can contact the hospital chaplain or the minister of their choice to discuss the form of the service and how it can best articulate their feelings and meet their needs. Other parents may prefer to organise a personal ceremony, at home or in some place that carries meaning for them.

Some parents organise a memorial ceremony every year, on the anniversary of their baby's birth or death. Some hospital chaplains hold monthly memorial services in the hospital chapel. Bereaved parents can attend these whenever they wish and on special dates such as anniversaries.

Some hospitals hold one special annual memorial service to which all bereaved parents are invited. Some parish churches hold annual memorial services which all bereaved parents can attend.

Other memorials

There are many other public or private ways in which parents may choose to create memorials to their babies. Some parents will know very clearly what they want; some may find it helpful to know what other parents have done.

Some examples are -

- having framed photographs of the baby, or a framed painting taken from a photograph

- making a scrapbook of everything to do with the pregnancy and the baby's life and death. For example, the slip of paper confirming the pregnancy, any test results, the hospital cooperation card, photographs of the mother pregnant, a photograph of the scan, any other photographs, pictures by siblings, a letter to the baby, a poem, the baby's cot card and name band if the baby died after birth, cards and letters people sent, a photograph of the cemetery or the baby's grave, and so on.

- pressing a posy of flowers from the baby's funeral and making these into a memento

- putting flowers on the baby's grave (where this is permitted, see page 65) on anniversaries and other important dates.

- buying a small vase, possibly cut glass or silver, with the baby's name engraved on it, and putting flowers in this on special anniversaries or whenever the parents feel the need to grieve

- visiting a special place on anniversaries

- sending flowers or some other gift to, for example, a hospital or old people's home on anniversaries, so meeting parents' need to grieve and enabling them to bring pleasure to other people at the same time

- entering their baby's name in a baby book of remembrance in their local church or other place of worship

- planting a tree or ornamental shrub in a favourite place or in the cemetery where the baby is buried

- putting up a bench with a memorial plaque in a well-loved place or in the cemetery where the baby is buried.

It may be important to remind parents that it is never too late to commemorate and show their love and grief for their baby. It need not be done at the time of the baby's death.

SUPPORT FOR PROFESSIONALS

Difficulties faced by professionals

Giving care and support to parents whose baby is dying or has died is extremely demanding, difficult and stressful. As well as feeling for, and with, the parents, professionals also have to cope with their own feelings. They have to do this at the same time as giving medical and practical care.

Difficulties can include -

- painful feelings. All professionals feel distressed and saddened when a baby dies. All feel for the parents and to some extent share the parents' sense of loss. Many professionals are reminded of their own experiences of loss and may then feel especially sad or find it particularly hard to cope.

- a sense of having failed, because a baby has died. There may also be feelings of guilt or anger. Professionals sometimes blame themselves, or a colleague, or even the parents. In some circumstances, they may fear litigation.

- stress and exhaustion. Caring for dying babies and bereaved people is difficult and tiring and it is not always possible to take time to recuperate. Pressure which can be tolerated in normal circumstances can become intolerable when there is additional emotional stress. It is particularly stressful to work without clear guidelines, or with procedures which seem to minimise the emotional significance of the event.

- feelings of helplessness and frustration. Many professionals are acutely aware that they cannot provide what parents most want and need: they cannot bring back

...e pregnancy which has ended or the baby who has died.

...heightened awareness of personal fears (especially fear of ...eath) and conflicts.

The need for support

...professionals are to provide parents with the quality of care ...at they need, it is essential that they themselves have ...ccess to appropriate support. This applies to *all* ...rofessionals. It applies to professionals working in the ...ommunity as well as those in hospital; and to all levels and ...isciplines.

Support should be available to professionals *as a matter of course*. It should be built into the system within which ...ey work.

The kind and degree of support that is needed will vary ...om person to person and from case to case. So it is ...mportant that different kinds of support are available for ...dividuals to use as they need.

...rofessionals involved in the care and support of bereaved ...arents need -

...to recognise, and to receive recognition from managers ...nd colleagues, that they are doing a difficult job which ...makes special demands over and above their professional ...xpertise; and that therefore if they need support, it is not ...ecause of either professional or personal inadequacy.

...to be equipped with relevant knowledge, skills and ...nderstanding

...to feel confident that they (and colleagues) are providing ...adequate and appropriate care

...the knowledge that they are working as part of a team with ...shared standards and aims

...opportunities to express their own feelings and needs.

The death of a baby is one of the most painful experiences any parent can suffer. It is also painful for the staff to come close to these parents and to witness their grief.

(Jenni Thomas, Counsellor, Wycombe General Hospital Maternity Unit and SCBU)

Units need a regular forum where each perinatal death is discussed, so that information and awareness are concerted (a safety net for patients); and where sharing of experiences promotes the welfare and clinical knowledge of doctors and nurses (a safety net for staff).

(Bourne S and Lewis E, *'Pregnancy after stillbirth and neonatal death'*, The Lancet, 7 July 1984, 31-3)

Support for professionals: recommendations

● All professionals caring for bereaved parents should feel confident about their own ability to give appropriate, understanding care. Basic, post-basic and in-service training should be provided on bereavement and grief after the loss of a baby, and on the skills needed to help bereaved parents. It is especially important that staff develop the ability to listen.

● All professionals working with bereaved parents should feel assured that they are working within an operational policy which is adequate and appropriate.

Each hospital and each health authority should have a clear and detailed policy for the management of miscarriage, stillbirth and neonatal death, and this policy should be shared and understood by all staff involved.

Professionals should have opportunities to influence policy and improve practice on the basis of their experience of caring for bereaved parents.

● The provision of support for professionals should be a part of policy and integrated into day-to-day practice. There is a need for -

- an open and supportive atmosphere in which staff can share problems with each other and talk about their feelings, so helping each other in informal ways

- more formal opportunities for staff to share experiences and discuss their feelings about or problems with particular cases, away from the wards

- opportunities for staff to talk confidentially to someone (such as a bereavement counsellor) individually if they wish, in a private, comfortable place. They may want to discuss worries about a particular case; or their own feelings.

- agreed strategies to help alleviate stress, eg management of time and tasks so that staff are able to recover from a death before moving on to their next patient/client; regular appraisal with opportunities to discuss any difficulties; opportunities for positive feedback from colleagues and also from bereaved parents.

Senior staff have a particular responsibility to watch for signs of strain or difficulty among staff; and to facilitate discussion. They also need to be aware of their own needs for support.

Responsibilities should be shared as much as possible. It may benefit parents if one member of staff is mainly responsible for their care, but the same professional should not be asked to care for all bereaved parents.

All professionals caring for bereaved parents need to feel that they are working as part of a team and do not bear sole responsibility. Within the team, it may be necessary to recognise and coordinate members' different skills.

All those who support bereaved parents need to be well informed about procedures and arrangements, about the choices open to parents, and about sources of information, help and advice. They need to feel able to answer parents' questions confidently, and to meet their needs adequately.

Professionals can obtain information and/or support from many of the organisations listed on page 78.

Part of the commitment to improve services to bereaved parents is the care and support of the professionals who are looking after them. We have arranged workshops for all staff to which medical staff and hospital chaplains are invited and we hope that we will learn from the sharing of experiences and discussion of problems, as this in turn will benefit the mothers and fathers in our care.

(Bhattacharjee C, *'Improving the care of bereaved parents'* Nursing Standard, 21 February 1990, Vol 4, No 22, 18-20)

SOURCES AND FURTHER READING

Alderson P, *Saying goodbye to your baby* , (a leaflet for parents), Stillbirth and Neonatal Death Society, London 1986

Batcup G, Clarke J P and Purdie D W, *'Disposal arrangements for fetuses lost in the second trimester',* British Journal of Obstetrics and Gynaecology , Vol 95, pp 547 - 550, June 1988

Bourne S and Lewis E, '*Pregnancy after stillbirth and neonatal death: Psychological risks and management',* The Lancet , pp 31 - 33, 7 July 1984

Borg S and Lasker J, *When pregnancy fails,* Routledge Kegan Paul, London 1983

British Institute of Funeral Directors, *Funerals for fetal remains* , 1986

Enkin M, Keirse M J N C and Chalmers I, *A guide to effective care in pregnancy and childbirth* , Oxford University Press, Oxford, 1989

Forrest G C, Standish E, and Baum J D, *'Support after perinatal death: A study of support and counselling after perinatal death',* British Medical Journal , Vol 285, pp 1475 - 1479, 20 Nov 1982
See also the letter replying to the above article: Bourne S and Lewis E., British Medical Journal , Vol 286, 8 Jan 1983

Friedman T, '*Women's experiences of general practitioner management of miscarriage',* Journal of the Royal College of General Practitioners , Vol 39, pp 456 - 458, Nov 1989

Hey V, Itzin C, Saunders L and Speakman M A, (eds), *Hidden loss - Miscarriage and ectopic pregnancy* , The Women's Press, London 1989

Huisjes H J, *Spontaneous abortion* , Churchill Livingstone, Edinburgh 1984

Hutti M H, *'A quick reference table of interventions to assist families to cope with pregnancy loss or neonatal death'*, Birth , 15:1, pp 33 - 35, March 1988, Berkeley, USA

Joint Committee for Hospital Chaplaincy, *Miscarriage, stillbirth and neonatal death: Guidelines in pastoral care for clergy and hospital chaplaincy* , London 1987

Kohner N and Henley A, *'When a baby dies. The experience of late miscarriage, stillbirth and neonatal death'*, Pandora Press, London, to be published late 1991

Lewis E and Bourne S, *'Perinatal death,'* Bailliere's Clinical Obstretrics and Gynaecology , Vol 3, No 4, pp 935 - 953, December 1989

Lewis E and Bryan E M, *'Management of perinatal loss of a twin',* British Medical Journal , Vol 297, pp 1321 - 1323, 19 Nov 1988.

Lovell A, 'Some questions of identity: Late miscarriage, stillbirth and perinatal loss', Social Science and Medicine , Vol 17, No 11, pp 755 - 761, 1983

McIntosh N and Eldridge C, 'Neonatal loss: The neglected side of neonatal care', Archives of Disease in Childhood, Vol 59, pp 585 - 587, 1984

Moulder C, Miscarriage: Women's experiences and needs, Pandora Press, London, 1990

Oakley A, McPherson A and Roberts H, Miscarriage, Penguin, London 1990 (revised from 1984 Fontana edition)

Peppers L and Knapp R, Motherhood and mourning, Praeger, 1980

Royal College of Obstetricians and Gynaecologists, Report on the management of perinatal deaths, London, October 1985

SATFA, Support after termination for abnormality - Handbook for parents, Satfa, 29-30 Soho Square, London W1V 6JB

Wells R, Helping children cope with grief, Sheldon Press, London 1988

USEFUL ADDRESSES

Support for parents

The Stillbirth and Neonatal Death Society (SANDS)
28 Portland Place
London W1N 4DE
071 436 5881

For parents whose babies are born dead or die soon after birth.

The Miscarriage Association (MA)
PO Box 24
Ossett
West Yorkshire WF5 9XG
(Most weekday mornings: 0924 264579, Answerphone: 0924 830515)

For parents who have experienced miscarriage.

The Twins and Multiple Births Association (TAMBA)
For parents who have lost one or both twins, or babies from a multiple birth. Contact through SANDS (see above).

BLISSLINK
17-21 Emerald Street
London WC1N 3QL
071 831 9393

For parents of babies in intensive and special care including bereaved parents.

NIPPERS Bereavement Group
c/o Sam Segal Perinatal Unit
St Mary's Hospital
Praed Street
London W2 1NY
071 725 1487

For bereaved parents of premature babies and babies in special care.

Support After Termination For Abnormality (SATFA)
29-30 Soho Square
London W1V 6JB
071 439 6124

For parents who have had or may have a pregnancy terminated because of their baby's abnormality.

The National Childbirth Trust (NCT)
Alexandra House
Oldham Terrace
Acton
London W3 6NH
081 992 8637

Most branches can put parents in touch with others who have had a similar experience and many have a miscarriage support group.

The Foundation for the Study of Infant Deaths (FSID)
35 Belgrave Square
London SW1X 8PS
071 235 0965

The Scottish Cot Deaths Trust
c/o Mrs Hazel Brooke
Royal Hospital for Sick Children
Yorkhill
Glasgow G3 8SJ
041 357 3946

for parents whose babies have died as a result of Sudden Infant Death Syndrome (cot death or SIDS).

British Association for Counselling
37a Sheep Street
Rugby
Warwickshire CV2 3BX
0788 78328/9
Information on where to get counselling locally.

Relate
Hubert Gray College
Little Church Street
Rugby
Warwickshire CV21 3AP
0788 73241
Confidential counselling for relationship problems of any kind. Local branches under Relate in the phone book.

Queries on certification and registration

Registrar General for England and Wales
St Catherine's House
10 Kingsway
London WC2B 6JP
071 242 0262

Registrar General for Northern Ireland
Oxford House
49-55 Chichester Street
Belfast BT1 4HL
0232 235 211

Registrar General for Scotland
General Register Office
New Register House
Edinburgh EH1 3YT
031 334 0380

SANDS wishes to thank all members of the working party whose discussions and contributions form the substance of this booklet:

Gill Mallinson, SANDS Adviser (Chair)

Pat Atkinson, Norfolk Bereavement Care

British Association for Perinatal Medicine:
Richard Pearse, Consultant Neonatal Paediatrician

British Institute of Funeral Directors:
David Hampton, Funeral Director
Mark Tyack, Funeral Director

British Paediatric Association:
Keith Dodd, Consultant Paediatrician

Gillian Gau, Consultant Perinatal Pathologist

Joan Greenwood, Nursing Officer Midwifery,
Department of Health (Observer)

Health Visitors' Association:
Ros Meek, Professional Liaison Officer

Institute of Burial and Cremation Administration:
Jon Luby, IBCA Adviser

Joint Committee for Hospital Chaplaincy:
Neville Smith, Chaplain, Guy's Hospital

Miscarriage Association:
Christine Moulder, Honorary Research Fellow, Sussex University
Kathryn Ladley, Past Secretary

National Association of Funeral Directors:
Pat Bennett, Funeral Director
John Lodge, Funeral Director

National Childbirth Trust:
Mary Davies, Co-ordinator for Miscarriage Information and Support

Royal College of General Practitioners:
Michael Carmi, Associate Adviser in General Practice
Mairi Scott, General Practitioner

Royal College of Midwives:
Greta Balfour, Senior Professional Officer

Royal College of Nursing:
Vicki Nix, Midwifery Adviser

Royal College of Obstetricians and Gynaecologists:
Gaye Henson, Consultant Obstetrician

Society of Registration Officers:
Norman Stephens, Superintendent Registrar

Stillbirth and Neonatal Death Society:
Maureen Edmondson, SANDS Member
Eimear Mallen, Former SANDS Executive Member
Julie Ransley, SANDS Vice-Chair

SANDS wishes to thank the following organisations whose valuable financial assistance has made the production of this book possible

King Edward's Hospital Fund for London

Littlewoods Organisation plc

Wyeth Nutrition, supported by an educational grant

Smith's Charity

The Hon Michael Astor's 1969 Charitable Trust

Scottish Home and Health Department

SANDS thanks the many professionals and parents who contributed photographs and the examples of good practice and personal experiences on which these Guidelines are based.

Printed with the support of British Telecom